Practice Development in Community Nursing

Principles and processes

WITHDRAWN

Edited by

Rosamund M Bryar PhD, MPhil, BNurs, RN, RHV, NDN Cert, RM, Cert Ed (FE)
Professor of Community and Primary Car⋯⋯⋯ City University, London, UK

and

U0774193

Jane M Griffiths PhD, BNurs, RGN, NDN Cert
Lecturer in Community Nursing, University of Manchester, Manchester, UK

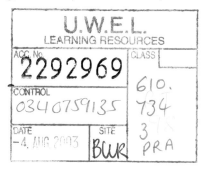

ARNOLD

A member of the Hodder Headline Group
LONDON

This first edition published in 2003 by Arnold,
a member of the Hodder Headline Group,
338 Euston Road, London NW1 3BH

http://www.arnoldpublishers.com

Distributed in the USA by
Oxford University Press Inc.,
198 Madison Avenue, New York, NY10016
Oxford is a registered trademark of Oxford University Press

Whilst the advice and information in this book are believed to be true and
accurate at the date of going to press, neither the authors nor the publisher
can accept any legal responsibility or liability for any errors or omissions
that may be made. In particular (but without limiting the generality of the
preceding disclaimer) every effort has been made to check drug dosages;
however, it is still possible that errors have been missed. Furthermore,
dosage schedules are constantly being revised and new side-effects
recognized. For these reasons the reader is strongly urged to consult the
drug companies' printed instructions before administering any of the drugs
recommended in this book.

British Library Cataloguing in Publication Data
A catalogue record for this book is available from the British Library

Library of Congress Cataloging-in-Publication Data
A catalog record for this book is available from the Library of Congress

ISBN 0 340 75913 5

1 2 3 4 5 6 7 8 9 10

Commissioning Editor: Georgina Bentliff
Development Editor: Heather Smith
Project Editor: Wendy Rooke
Production Controller: Lindsay Smith
Cover Design: Amina Dudhia

Typeset in 10/12pt Minion by Phoenix Photosetting, Chatham, Kent
Printed and bound in Malta

What do you think about this book? Or any other Arnold title?
Please send your comments to feedback.arnold@hodder.co.uk
http://www.arnoldpublishers.com

This book is dedicated to all the staff of the former community trusts in Hull and East Yorkshire with thanks for the inspiration, challenges and support they gave us both.

Contents

Contributors

Katrina Bannigan BD BSc SROT

Katrina Bannigan is a Senior Lecturer in Research Methods, School of Health and Social Care, University of Teesside. Prior to this she worked as a research and development occupational therapist at the Institute of Rehabilitation, Hull and East Yorkshire Hospitals NHS Trust. This role involved being the lead for research and development in occupational therapy and studying for her PhD at the University of Hull. Her PhD focused on increasing the use of research findings in four allied health professions (dietetics, occupational therapy, physiotherapy and speech and language therapy). Her thesis was closely related to the development aspect of her work, which involved developing evidence-based practice within the occupational therapy department in the trust. This involved leading the work on clinical governance, training therapists in critical appraisal skills, leading journal clubs, evaluating the service and working with individual and groups of therapists to facilitate the use of research-based knowledge in routine clinical practice. Nationally she has published articles and presented conference papers about evidence-based practice and clinical governance. She is particularly interested in the role of managers in increasing the use of research findings in practice development.

Rosamund Bryar PhD, MPhil, BNurs, RN, RHV, NDN Cert, RM, Cert Ed (FE)

Rosamund Bryar is Professor of Community and Primary Care Nursing, City University, London. Between 1995 and 2000 she held the chair of Community Healthcare Nursing Practice at the University of Hull and was professional lead for health visiting in Hull and Holderness Community Health NHS Trust. Throughout her career she has been concerned with the development of different aspects of primary health care services, and for 3 years was part of Teamcare Valleys, the South Wales Valleys primary health care development unit. Her research interests are concerned with the barriers to effective primary health care practice; chronic disease management; and the process by which practitioners develop research skills. She is joint editor with Professor Sally Kendall of *Primary Health Care Research and Development*. In 2002 she was appointed as a member of the NICE Appraisal Committee.

S. José Closs BSc (Hons), RGN, MPhil, PhD

S. José Closs was appointed as Professor of Nursing Research at the University of Leeds in January 2000. She has been an active researcher for 20 years in various posts at the universities of Nottingham, Edinburgh, Hull and then Leeds. She has an interest in clinical nursing activities, including: sleep and pain management, particularly in older people; discharge planning; and the implementation of research findings. She has published widely in all these areas. Building on this work she is developing an interest in interdisciplinary research and research implementation, with colleagues from medicine, pharmacy, radiography and others.

Jo Cooke BNurs, RGN, RHV, MA

Jo Cooke holds a community qualification and, during the time of the study reported in this book, held a joint appointment between Community Health Sheffield and the School of Health and Related Research (ScHARR) at the University of Sheffield. Since that time Jo has worked on an Association of Directors of Social Services initiative, based at the Dartington Social Research Unit and the University of Sheffield, promoting evidence-based practice in social care. Currently in Sheffield, Jo works as a research co-ordinator with the primary care research network Trent Focus, which involves the Universities of Sheffield, Nottingham and Leicester. Trent Focus aims to support R&D in primary care, and Jo has particular responsibilities for developing research capacity at the interface with social care.

Joanne Dorsman RN, RM, RHV, BSc (Hons), BA (Hons), Adv Dip

Joanne Dorsman trained initially as a registered nurse and midwife and gained extensive experience in gynaecological nursing before qualifying as a health visitor. In 1997 she took up a health visitor appointment with the integrated health visiting and district nursing team at Middleton Nursing Development Unit, and a year later became joint clinical leader. During the 3-year period as clinical leader, Jo was actively involved in leading a number of community-based public health initiatives, including co-ordinating the planning process for a successful third-wave Sure Start bid. She recently moved to her present post as Sure Start Project Co-ordinator for Health at Avondale Health Centre in Bolton, a Sure Start area where she is pursuing her broad interests in public health.

Kate Gerrish, PhD, MSc, BNurs, RGN, RM, NDN Cert

Kate Gerrish is Professor of Nursing Practice Development, School of Nursing and Midwifery, University of Sheffield and the Sheffield Teaching Hospitals NHS Trust. She has held a variety of posts in community and hospital-based nursing practice and nurse education in the UK and Zambia. Her research interests span the areas of transcultural nursing, nursing development and nurse education, and she has published widely in each of these areas. Kate has a long-standing interest in practice development and for several years has been a member of the Practice Development Accreditation Panel of the University of Leeds. She is joint editor, with Dr James Nazroo, of the journal *Ethnicity and Health*.

Hilary Gledhill RN

Hilary Gledhill is a registered nurse who qualified in 1983. At the time of writing she was employed as the ward manager at Hornsea Cottage Hospital, a position she held for 10 years. During her time there Hilary developed a keen interest in practice development and managing change within a clinical area. Hilary is now employed by the

Yorkshire Coast and Wolds Primary Care Trust as professional nurse lead and clinical governance co-ordinator. This new and challenging role enables her to take a lead in developing the infrastructure to deliver the clinical governance agenda in this new organization while still retaining a front-line approach to practice development within the Minor Injury Units and community hospitals within the Primary Care Trust.

Jane Griffiths PhD, BNurs, RGN, NDN Cert

Jane Griffiths is a lecturer in community nursing at the University of Manchester. She leads the district nursing pathway of the Community Specialist Practitioner degree, where there is a strong emphasis on both evidence-based practice and practice development. Before going to Manchester in 1998 she held a position in practice development in East Yorkshire, where she was professional lead for district nursing and lecturer in the University of Hull. As lead district nurse she became interested in guideline implementation and audit as a means of developing evidence-based district nursing practice. It was in this post that the need for a book such as this became apparent. Her interest in developing practice in district nursing came from her research experience as a research assistant and then a PhD student at Liverpool University. Her doctoral dissertation was an ethnographic study of district nursing work which described the culture of district nursing with particular emphasis on the factors that hindered optimal practice. She has produced several publications on practice development derived from her doctoral research, research into barriers to research implementation and an audit of care plan evaluations in district nursing. Between 1996 and 2002 she was a member of the Queen's Nursing Institute Practice Development and Research Committee.

Andrew Leeming BSc, MA

Andrew Leeming is currently a senior consultant within Enterprise PLC, a company specializing in community economic development and regeneration, which works in particular with the local authority sector. Prior to this he was a Community Development Worker for Stockport NHS Trust for 5 years, having previously worked in health promotion in Nottingham. A masters in health promotion enabled him to start analysing some of the practical conflicts arising from evaluating his own working practice and allowed him to consider these issues in greater detail than is usually possible in our normal working practice. His move into the wider public arena via his work with Enterprise has allowed him to constantly refine and remodel his evaluative practice and share his expertise with others. Currently involved in the new modernization agenda for local government, which has a strong focus on the community, the challenge is to find the right evaluation tools to demonstrate and pick out areas of worth and importance for future development.

Joyce L. Marshall RN, RM, BSc (Hons), MPH

Joyce L. Marshall is a researcher at the Mother and Infant Research Unit, University of Leeds. When the research that forms the basis of the chapter was carried out, she was based at the Centre for Research in Primary Care in Leeds. She currently has a regional NHS R&D Fellowship award and is conducting research on the way research 'evidence' is used in midwifery and health visiting practice – in particular, how research knowledge is understood and used within the context of the clinical encounter. Her clinical background is in midwifery and in the past she has worked in public health and primary care research and primary care development. She has a special interest in public health issues, particularly in relation to mother and child health.

Jane Mischenko BSc (Hons), MA, RGN, RHV

Jane Mischenko held the post of practice development lead within the Middleton Nursing Development Unit in Leeds at the time of writing the chapter, and has now taken up a post as a clinical development facilitator for community nurses in the Leeds Community and Mental Health Trust. Her professional background was initially general nursing in an acute trust and then, more recently, health visiting. She has a particular interest in the development of the public health approach to health visiting.

Linda Pearson BSc, RN, PhD, PGCE (FE)

Linda Pearson is a freelance 'development facilitator' currently working as a distance learning tutor for the Royal College of Nursing Institute. She registered as a nurse in 1980 as part of a BSc/RN course in Liverpool University and has worked in a range of posts, within and outside of nursing, ever since. In the 1980s she gained a PhD in Dental Sciences and has brought this interest to her research into aspects of nurse- and carer-delivered mouth care. She has had a number of lecturing posts in nursing departments and has developed partnerships with practitioners in the UK and overseas in order to explore and understand practice issues. She has a long-standing interest into what facilitates personal, professional and community development. This began through working in a Primary Health Care Clinic in Jamaica at the beginning of the 1990s. In 1997 she discovered participatory appraisal (PA), and her ongoing association with a health-related project in an inner city estate in Hull has affirmed her belief in the approach.

Nicki Whitfield RGN, NDN Cert, BSc (Hons) Nursing Studies

Nicki Whitfield gained experience of hospital nursing before taking up a community nursing post and subsequently qualifying as a district nurse. She worked at Middleton Nursing Development Unit (NDU) in Leeds from 1993 when it was first accredited, becoming joint clinical leader in 1998. She has recently taken up a new position as Clinical Development Facilitator for District Nursing for the south Leeds area and Tissue Viability Nurse working with the city-wide Tissue Viability Service, which covers the community nursing, mental health, learning disabilities and nursing home sectors. Her interest in practice development evolved from involvement in the NDU and the belief that district nurses should consider the health needs of the local population, not just those of individual clients registered on a caseload.

Forewords

Nursing has a central part to play in the care and health of individuals, families and communities. To help achieve high-quality nursing care, attention needs to be paid to the processes and support systems in place to facilitate the development of nurses and nursing. In the 1990s I was Director of Nursing in Hull and Holderness Community Health NHS Trust. Professional leadership for all nursing disciplines in the Trust was provided by a lead practitioner in each discipline. I was concerned that this professional leadership should be practice based and also informed by academic input from the University of Hull, where the local school of nursing was located. Each of the professional leads had a practice remit to help ensure that any developments they initiated or led were relevant to the practitioners and communities using the service. This practice base helped ensure local relevance of the practice development agenda, but I also thought it was important that practice development in the Hull and East Riding area be informed by, and inform, the wider practice development arena. I therefore sought and obtained support for two new posts funded by the NHS: a Chair and Lecturer in Community Healthcare Nursing Practice. The Chair was also professional lead for health visiting; it had a practice remit and was located in my Trust, and the Lecturer was professional lead for district nursing in the adjacent East Yorkshire Community NHS Trust.

This book has arisen from the experience of the first two post holders of the lack of readily available guidance on practice development in community nursing. The book contains chapters giving real-life practice development experience and draws on many additional examples of practice development initiatives. The practice examples are underpinned by theory and contribute to the extension of knowledge about successful approaches to practice development. In my view this book provides evidence of the value of joint NHS–university appointments which enable the identification of practice issues that can then be explored and responded to by academic methods, such as new courses, research, publications or other activities. I anticipate that this book will be of use to all nurses working in community and primary care settings, who are constantly seeking to extend and develop their practice. Production of this book reinforces my original vision that these NHS–university professional lead posts would contribute both to local and national practice development.

Malcolm Anderson RMN, RN
Formerly Director of Nursing,
Hull and Holderness Community Health NHS Trust

As we enter a new millennium, change is upon us. Health care practice and styles of delivery are on an edge of major explosion of new ideas and knowledge. Through this knowledge health care is becoming more complex; this produces an exciting challenge for all in nursing.

The potential of scientific experimentation will impact on society at large and widen the opportunities available to each of us on how our health care dilemmas are managed. We are moving away from the industrial era into a digital world where the sharing of knowledge is no longer problematic for those who want to learn. Communication opportunities are more varied, transparent and fast.

Although the nursing knowledge base is growing, like other clinical groups, disseminating this knowledge alone currently has little effect on clinical practice. The expectation of good clinical governance requires this situation to change.

Members of today's society have high expectations of their health care system. There are also clear expectations for nursing delivery. I believe nursing has a special place in this changing scenario. We need to be seen applying the science of evidence-based care while recognizing the importance and protecting the art of care giving. We, as nurses, will need to be willing to continue clinical learning throughout our professional lives and be willing to change. To deliver the requirements of good nursing we must consistently remind ourselves of the core principles of nursing: be patient, focused, promote good practice and prevent poor, unethical care.

Nursing leadership to support this change comes in various guises. The contributors to this book, leaders within their own spheres of nursing, provide for us, through the various chapters, a window on how we can move forward. The book focuses on the important and largely unrecognized development role of community nursing, but it has important messages for all nurses, irrespective of their area of work.

Alexandra Henderson RN, RM, RHV, BSc Nursing (Hons)
Director of Nursing, East Riding and Hull Community NHS Trust

Acknowledgements

This book is underpinned by our experiences over more than 20 years in practice development activities. During this time we have worked with and learnt from innumerable people who have helped develop our understanding of practice development: we extend our thanks to them all. The contributors to this book have been more than helpful and we thank them for their interest in this project. We are very grateful to Malcolm Anderson and Alex Henderson for agreeing to write the forewords. Alex was director of nursing in East Yorkshire Community NHS Trust and Malcolm Anderson was director of nursing in Hull and Holderness Community Health NHS Trust. We would like to acknowledge the part that their commitment to practice development made to our ideas about the development of practice.

Ros would like to thank her brother, Quentin, his wife, Siobhan, their children, Saoirse and Laurence, and her aunt and uncle, Muriel and Gordon Robertson, for their support, encouragement and tolerance during the preparation of this book. She would also like to thank other family members and friends for their support. Ashma Ponniah and Caroline White, secretaries in the Public Health and Primary Care Unit, City University have provided invaluable help in getting the final manuscript ready. She thanks them and the other members of staff of the Unit for their forbearance. Bounty and Pookie have provided wonderful companionship and their need for walks during the preparation of this book has been therapeutic!

Jane would like to thank her husband Peter for his wonderful support, her daughter Annaruth and baby daughter Isabelle who was born during the preparation of this book. She would also like to thank her parents Shirley and Geoff for their endless support and encouragement, and Monica and Wendy for being a constant source of inspiration. She would like to thank Ann Handy for her unerring belief in possibilities and the many friends and colleagues who have supported, encouraged and challenged her over the years.

1

Introduction

Rosamund Bryar and Jane Griffiths

Purpose of this chapter

- To discuss the need for a book about practice development in community nursing.
- To discuss the purpose of the book.
- To explain what we mean by practice development.
- To explain the importance of practice development in community nursing.
- To introduce the sections of the book.
- To suggest how the book could be used.

WHY DO WE NEED THIS BOOK?

The practice of nurses and health visitors working in community and primary care settings is continually changing and developing. For example, district nurses now care for people with highly specialized needs and carry out technical care such as flushing central lines, Doppler ultrasound assessment and compression bandaging; practice nurses provide advice on immunizations and health care for people travelling to far-flung parts of the world; those caring for people with mental health needs have seen enormous changes in their work with the closure of the long-stay psychiatric hospitals; and health visitors, in particular, have an important public health remit.

Set these developments in the wider policy context of developments such as Primary Medical Services pilots/contracts and Walk-In Centres, Health and Education Action Zones, Primary Care Trusts (PCTs) and their equivalents in Northern Ireland, Scotland and Wales (*see* Note 1), Health Improvement and Modernization Programmes, Nurse Prescribing, NHS Direct, Intermediate Care, Integrated Nursing Teams, and Teaching PCT's, and you have a hotbed for change. All of these changes have required nurses and health visitors to gain knowledge in different areas of practice, to learn new skills, to work with new team members, and to implement new communication systems: in short to develop their practice. The publication of the *Scope of Professional Practice* in 1992 (UKCC, 1992) permitted nurses to extend their practice and develop their roles according to the requirements of clients and the service, and released the straightjacket on nursing practice. The updated *Code of Professional Conduct*, published by the Nursing and Midwifery Council in 2002, reinforces this approach. In addition, the NHS modernization plan places emphasis on the development of nurses and nursing as part of the process of refocusing on high-quality clinical care (Department of Health, 1999, 2000, 2001a). Clinical nurses working in primary health care now have key positions on PCT executive boards and have a direct impact on the configuration of primary, secondary and tertiary services in their area. Future scanning suggests that the roles that nurses hold in primary health care will become more and more important as nurses (and other practitioners) take on more of the first contact activity within primary health care and develop their roles to meet the needs of their local populations (Wanless, 2002). Such changes provide nurses and health visitors with unprecedented opportunities for service and practice development.

However, much development work goes on unrecorded in isolated pockets nationally as part of the everyday work of professional development groups, professional leads, practice development co-ordinators and facilitators. For the majority of these people, the purpose of change is to improve practice and the quality of services provided for the community. They are involved in the change process and have little time to consider disseminating the steps that they went through to bring about changes. As the National Co-ordinating Centre for NHS Service Delivery and Organization R&D (2001:5) reports:

> We already know that managers and professionals are keen to learn from research and to base their decisions on evidence. However, substantial numbers of managers and clinical professionals argue much of the evidence about effective change management is located in the heads of practitioners and has yet to find its way into the scholarly journals.

Lessons that they have learnt about the process of development are therefore lost to the wider community nursing world. These practitioners certainly have less incentive to disseminate information about the work they are involved with than their academic colleagues. Researchers in community nursing have an incentive to publish and disseminate their findings in the terms of their contracts and in the form of the research assessment exercise (*see* Note 2). As part of this process academics have an incentive to network with colleagues in other universities and the health service to develop and submit proposals for research funding. Nurses working in development posts have less of an imperative to network with colleagues and disseminate their findings: their focus is on securing local change. They may also have less time, as these activities are not necessarily seen as an important component of their role. Publication and dissemination is clearly important, however, so that good practice can be shared, and time spent starting from scratch and making mistakes avoided or reduced.

In 1995 we were appointed to two innovative posts in community trusts in Hull and East Yorkshire. In these posts we held academic appointments as the Professor and Lecturer in Community Healthcare Nursing Practice and trust appointments as professional leads respectively in health visiting (RB) and district nursing (JG). As professional leads we had the remit to develop practice in our disciplines and to contribute to the overall development agenda within the nursing and other disciplines in the trusts. When we came into post we began to look around for some guidance on models and methods of developing practice in community nursing, but found that there was a dearth of information on this subject aimed at community nurses. This lack provided the motivation for the current book, which aims to inform the process of development of community and primary care nursing.

There also seemed to be a need for such a book for practitioners undertaking community specialist practitioner qualifications, who were being urged to consider how they would develop practice in their new roles. Again, there were no directly relevant textbooks available to these students to inspire them with ideas about what can be achieved in practice.

The purpose of the book therefore is to:

- Provide a discussion of definitions of practice and service development.
- Describe the theories underpinning practice and service development.
- To bring together accounts by community nurses and others of different approaches used to develop community nursing, to act as a resource for others involved in the development of community and primary care nursing.
- To provide a digest of resources providing additional information relevant to practice and service development.

The approach taken in this book is predicated on the goal of Health for All restated in Europe in *Health21* (World Health Organization, 1999:3): 'The one **constant goal** is to achieve full health potential for all.' To achieve this, four strategies for action are identified (World Health Organization, 1999:4):

- multisectoral strategies;
- outcome-driven programmes;
- integrated family- and community-orientated primary health care, supported by a flexible and responsive hospital system; and
- a participatory health development process that involves relevant partners for health, at all levels – home, school and worksite, local community and country – and that promotes joint decision making, implementation and accountability.

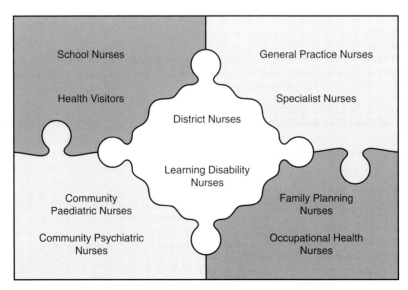

Fig. 1.1 *Community nurses*

Thus a wide definition of primary health care and community underpins this book (World Health Organization, 1999; Watson and Wilkinson, 2001; Cowley, 2002). An equally inclusive approach is taken to the issue of the audience for this book, whom we envisage as any nurse, health visitor or midwife working in a primary health care or community setting for all or part of their work. In the United Kingdom, we currently have a plethora of titles for people with a particular community remit, some of which are shown in Fig. 1.1. In practice, more and more nurses who have been traditionally hospital based are spending time in primary health care and community settings. It can be anticipated that this trend will continue to grow, contributing to the blurring of role definitions between nurses working in the community.

WHAT IS PRACTICE DEVELOPMENT?

Although we probably share a similar understanding of what is meant by practice, the meaning of development is less clear. The development arm of NHS research and development is often taken to mean applied research rather than developments that may draw on research methods, but are not research studies as such. In the context of this book we have adopted a far wider definition of development. Practice development is taken to mean a broad range of innovations that are initiated to improve practice and the services in which that practice takes place. We have used the term 'practice development' throughout to encompass practice *and service* development and sometimes also professional development. Examples of developments in practice, services and of professionals are provided in the second section of this book.

WHY IS THE DEVELOPMENT OF COMMUNITY NURSING IMPORTANT?

In the NHS research and development agenda, the focus has been on research with the development component frequently overlooked. With new posts in practice development and nurse consultant posts being initiated, and the importance of clinical governance emphasized for all practitioners, the development of practice, professionals and services has been brought to the fore. The NHS Plan (Department of Health, 2000) indicates that staff are keen to participate in the development of services:

> 9.24 Service modernisation relies on staff – especially those in clinical posts – having the time and space to redesign and re-organise their services. That is what staff throughout the NHS want to do. We will introduce 'service modernisation sessions' throughout the NHS where local managers and clinicians can apply the lessons that have been learned elsewhere in the NHS to redesign local services.

The publication of the NHS R&D strategy in 1991 (Department of Health, 1991) marked the beginning of widespread interest in knowledge-based practice. The need for knowledge-based practice in the NHS had been recognized at least two decades before in both nursing and medicine, but it was only in the 1990s that a strategic approach was developed to facilitate this process. Since then, a number of initiatives have been developed which support the collation of evidence, which may be used to develop health care practice. Enthusiasts for evidence-based practice initiated the Cochrane Collaboration to collate systematic reviews of available research evidence. In York, the Centre for Reviews and Dissemination was established to undertake systematic reviews, which are disseminated via the *Effective Health Care* bulletins. In the field of primary care, the National Primary Care Research and Development Centre was initiated in the mid-1990s to undertake research and contribute to the development agenda in primary care.

There are several reasons why development in community nursing is important. To begin with, most health care is undertaken in the community, so it is a very large and important sector of the health service, indeed Primary Care Trusts (PCTs) will, from 2002/3, account for management of 75 per cent of the NHS budget (Department of Health, 2001a). Another important consideration is that community nursing practice is, by its nature, hidden. Community nursing practitioners work in people's homes and other relatively isolated community settings that are often geographically quite separate from one another. Often, practice is not overseen by colleagues, as it might be in the acute hospital setting, and this can result in considerable variation in practice. Good practices can remain localized if neighbouring localities are unaware of what is happening nearby, and where practice is less than optimal, it may not be challenged if it is not overseen. An additional barrier is that it can be difficult to disseminate information to health centres and clinics which may be quite distant from libraries and other useful resources, and have, until recently or in some cases still, lacked access to IT resources.

Others also consider community practice an important area for development in moving towards more integrated services, suggesting:

> 3.4 A range of developments will offer possibilities for enhancing home-based care, for example health workers with an advocacy, mentoring and advisory role, internet-based advice, enhanced role for community pharmacists, patient-owned records and monitoring and other technologies based in the home environment.
>
> (Healthcare Panel, 2000:8)

New resources are now available to support development activities, including the Innovations web site (see Chapter 12); *Essence of Care* (Department of Health, 2001b), which provides a tool for benchmarking; the audit guide from the National Institute for Clinical Excellence (2002); lessons from nurse-led Personal Medical Services (PMS) pilots (Lewis, 2001); and the health visiting and school nurses development resource packs (Department of Health, 2001c, d). Development of practice and services is now enshrined in government policy, with health service quality a central tenet of the NHS Plan (Department of Health, 2000). There is a firm commitment to clinical governance from the government, which is being translated into practice locally by Primary Care Trusts. Practice and service development are firmly on the agenda of PCT boards. Indeed, development of services is now considered so important that the Foresight Healthcare Panel has suggested: '2.4 It is conceivable that the NHS in twenty years time will concentrate on the developmental aspects of health care . . .' (Healthcare Panel, 2000:7).

HOW IS THE BOOK STRUCTURED?

The book is divided into four sections. The first is concerned mainly with the theoretical underpinnings to practice and service development, the nature of evidence and the process of change. In the second section, examples are given of different approaches to the development of community nursing. The third section draws together the lessons from the first two sections and considers the ways ahead for the future development of community and primary care nursing. The final section provides a number of resources that may help to contribute to practice development activities. Each of the chapters begins with a statement of the purpose of the chapter, providing a learning guide for the reader. At the end of each chapter, the key points concerning practice development initiatives are summarized. Collectively these provide guidance on approaches that enhance the likelihood of achieving development in practice and services.

Section 1 begins with a discussion of the definitions of the various terms that are used in practice and service development. Chapter 2 clarifies the meaning of terms such as clinical effectiveness, implementation, dissemination and the 'D' component of NHS R&D. Many of the terms considered in this chapter are used interchangeably in practice and in the literature, leading to confusion both in understanding and application. The aim of this chapter is to provide clear definitions of these terms. The chapter also gives definitions of 'robust' evidence such as randomized controlled trials and systematic reviews, but also other sources of information that practitioners may draw upon in the absence of quality research evidence. The meaning of critical thinking and reflection are explored to this end. Finally the chapter takes a brief look at some recent developments in health services policy that have impacted on practice and service development, such as clinical governance, the National Institute for Clinical Excellence (NICE), the Commission for Health Improvement (CHI) and National Service Frameworks (NSFs).

The purpose of Chapter 3 is to examine the meaning of evidence in the practice of community nurses. All practice development initiatives may be considered to be attempts to apply the best current evidence to practice. However, there is wide debate about the nature of evidence and the quality of the available evidence. There is a lack of clarity in the literature about what is meant by evidence. This chapter considers these issues and explicates the term as applied to nursing, with particular reference to other types of evidence that nurses use in their day-to-day practice, such as personal knowledge and intuition.

Chapter 4 explores service and practice development in relation to the theory and processes of change. This chapter considers change at the level of the individual, team and organization. Different approaches to the introduction and management of change are considered, with practical examples drawn from community nursing and from multidisciplinary development projects. The complexity of change and the importance of the organizational context of the change are highlighted. In particular, strategies to increase the use of research in practice are considered.

The final chapter in this section looks at the importance of evaluation in practice development. Evaluation is a crucial part of any development in practice, but is sometimes overlooked. It can be carried out formatively throughout the development, to inform the direction of the project, or summatively at the end of the project to establish whether the development has been effective and should be disseminated or revised. Various approaches to evaluation are discussed, with particular emphasis on the developmental approach, which is used in community development work. Methods available to practitioners involved in evaluating projects are also discussed, some of which are applied in real examples in Section 2 of the book.

In Section 2, real examples are provided of approaches to practice development by practitioners and others. Examples are given of development activities which involved practice nurses, health visitors, school nurses, district nurses, community mental health nurses and others. The authors have provided honest accounts of their experiences of developing practice, reporting lessons learned and practical advice that can be tried in your own field of practice. All are concerned with the development process, but the emphasis in each is different. Some chapters are more concerned with practice, service or professional development. For example, Kate Gerrish, Joanne Dorsman, Nicki Whitfield and Jane Mischenko, in Chapter 10, provide a comprehensive literature review placing the Nursing Development Units movement in the context of wider changes in health care. In contrast, Linda Pearson, in Chapter 9, provides information on methods which practitioners can use, focusing on the professional development of practitioners to enable them to engage more effectively in community development. Throughout, the authors illustrate the types of skills needed to achieve effective practice development: negotiation skills, motivational skills, skills in appraising evidence, presentation skills, leadership skills and much patience and realism. As Kate Gerrish, Joanne Dorsman, Nicki Whitfield and Jane Mischenko note: Practice development takes time!

The authors are drawn from practice, academic and joint posts. When we were beginning to identify the people we would invite to contribute to this book we came up against the problem that we have discussed above: of the lack of publicly available information about developments in practice at that time. This situation has happily changed now; for example, with the introduction of the Beacon scheme (Department of Health, 2001e; *see* Chapter 12), the Innovations in health visiting and school nursing web site (*see* Chapter 12) and the development resource packs (Department of Health, 2001b, c). In the case of the practitioners, all speak from their own experiences. The academics also speak from their experiences of working closely with the practitioners involved in the development process.

In Chapter 6, Joyce Marshall gives a detailed account of her experience of facilitating the implementation of evidence-based guidelines in two general practices (in the context of a larger project), and the different approaches taken. Clinical guidelines are an important resource for practitioners seeking evidence to inform their practice. Joyce demonstrates how the dissemination of guidelines does not follow a linear path leading to implementation in practice. She compares the characteristics of one of the practices, where guideline implementation was successful, with the other practice, where it was less successful, and identifies the importance of the characteristics of the practice, i.e. the context of change. The work she describes used audit feedback as a mechanism for promoting change. She draws some useful conclusions for practitioners embarking upon similar work.

In Chapter 8, Jo Cooke uses the symbol of traffic lights as an approach to developing coping strategies in adolescent males at risk of self-harm, but also as an approach to practice development, i.e. stop, think, act. She used an action research approach to developing practice involving a repeating cycle of planning, development and evaluation. This chapter is one of several which demonstrates the involvement of people from other disciplines in practice development undertaken by community nurses. In Chapter 10, Kate Gerrish, Joanne Dorsman, Nicki Whitfield and Jane Mischenko describe the model of the Nursing Development Unit (NDU) as an approach to practice development. Like the other authors, they report the successes and failures of this approach and offer useful guidance for practitioners. The work of the Middleton NDU is described in the context of the literature on NDUs. The description of a number of developmental projects that the Unit has undertaken illustrates the potential of nursing teams to develop services by themselves or in collaboration with others. This chapter also illustrates that in many community nursing settings a number of development activities may be taking place at the same time.

In Chapter 7, Hilary Gledhill explores how barriers to developing and implementing evidence-based guidelines in two Minor Injuries Units were overcome using clinical supervision. She describes the process of this development in practice in detail and gives an honest account of the 'messiness' of the project, which, like many developments in practice, led to a series of spin-off projects. In Chapter 9, Linda Pearson offers a detailed, useable analysis of participatory appraisal as an approach to developing communities. In this rich account of the methods that she used, she gives examples of the wide range of tools that are available to facilitators to elicit information with and about the communities with which they are working.

In Section 3, the penultimate chapter of the book draws themes from the two earlier sections and addresses the lessons that can be learned about practice development in community nursing from the accounts and theory presented. Although there are differences in the approaches taken by the various authors, there are also many similarities, suggesting that although there might not be immutable rules about how to introduce change in practice, there are certain guiding principles.

Chapter 12, in Section 4, the final section of the book, contains information on access to the resources referred to in earlier sections. Additional resources are also included, which it is anticipated will support practice development activities and networking.

Some may question why this book is concerned 'only' with practice development in community nursing, rather than with multidisciplinary development. Within the huge primary health care development agenda, we believe that it is important to consider as much the uniprofessional as the multiprofessional development process. Our own experience has shown us that community nurses who have worked through the processes of development of their own services will be better placed to work with colleagues from other disciplines. For example, district nurses who have given thought to the assessment methods they use in the care of older people, and have developed their care in this area, will be in a better position to collaborate with colleagues from social services in joint service developments. Those looking for information on the wider development of primary health care are referred to the National Primary Care Development Team (*see* Chapter 12), Bryar and Bytheway (1996), Freeman *et al.* (1997), Pearson and Spencer (1997), Gabbay (1999), Iliffe and Lenihan (2001), Meads and Meads (2001), Unsworth (2001) as useful starting points.

HOW SHOULD YOU USE THIS BOOK?

This book does not need to be read from cover to cover. The chapters in the first section of the book may be read individually as essays in their own right, but are equally useful as the theoretical foundation for the examples from practice given in the second section of the book. The examples in section two can be dipped into according to your needs as practitioners or can be read as a whole as each of the authors has much to offer practitioners from other disciplines.

CONCLUSION

This introductory chapter has explained the origins of this book about practice development in community nursing and discussed the need for such a text for practitioners and students. Our use of the term 'practice development' has been clarified and the importance of practice development in community nursing in our current, receptive political climate explored. The various chapters of the book have been introduced and their relevance to the whole explained. Finally, suggestions have been made about how you might choose to use the book to assist you in your development work in practice.

Shifting the Balance of Power within the NHS – Securing Delivery (Department of Health, 2001a:24) asserts:

> 59. A real shift in the balance of power will not occur unless staff are empowered to make the necessary change. The cultural shift needed will, in many ways, be more crucial to the success of the project than new management structures. Staff need to be involved in decisions that effect service delivery. Empowerment comes when staff own the policies and are able to bring about real change.

We hope this book will provide a starting point for those seeking to bring about this real change in the practice, services and professional development of all nurses, health visitors and midwives working in primary health care.

REFERENCES

Bryar R and Bytheway B (Eds) 1996 *Changing Primary Health Care. The Teamcare Valleys Experience.* Blackwell Science, Oxford.

Cowley S (Ed) 2002 *Public Health in Policy and Practice. A Sourcebook for Health Visitors and Community Nurses.* Bailliere Tindall, Edinburgh.

Department of Health 1991 *Research for Health.* Department of Health, London.

Department of Health 1999 *Making a Difference: Strengthening the Nursing, Midwifery and Health Visiting Contribution to Health and Healthcare.* The Stationery Office, London.

Department of Health 2000 *The NHS Plan.* Department of Health, London.

Department of Health 2001a *Shifting the Balance of Power within the NHS – Securing Delivery.* Department of Health, London.

Department of Health 2001b *Essence of Care. Patient-focused Benchmarking for Health Care Practitioners.* Department of Health, London.

Department of Health 2001c *Health Visitor Practice Development Resource Pack.* The Health Visitor and School Nurse Development Programme. Department of Health, London.

Department of Health 2001d *School Nurse Practice Development Resource Pack.* The Health Visitor and School Nurse Development Programme. Department of Health, London.

Department of Health 2001e *NHS Beacons Programme Learning Handbook.* Department of Health, London.

Freeman R, Gillam S, Sherin C and Pratt J 1997 *Community Development and Involvement in Primary Health Care.* King's Fund, London.

Gabbay M (Ed) 1999 *The Evidence-Based Primary Care Handbook.* The Royal Society of Medicine Press Ltd, London.

Healthcare Panel 2000 *Health Care 2020.* Foresight. Department of Trade and Industry, London.

Iliffe S and Lenihan P 2001 Promoting primary care for older people in general practice using a community oriented approach. *Primary Health Care Research and Development* 2(2): 71–9.

Lewis R 2001 *Nurse-led Primary Care. Learning from PMS Pilots.* King's Fund, London.

Meads G and Meads T 2001 *Trust in Experience. Transferable Learning for Primary Care Trusts.* Radcliffe Medical Press, Abingdon.

National Co-ordinating Centre for NHS Service Delivery and Organisation R& D 2001 *Making Informed Decisions on Change. Key Points for Health Care Managers and Professionals.* NCCSDO, London School of Hygiene and Tropical Medicine, London.

National Institute for Clinical Excellence 2002 *Principles for Best Practice in Clinical Audit.* Radcliffe Medical Press, Abingdon.

Nursing and Midwifery Council 2002 *Code of Professional Conduct.* Nursing and Midwifery Council, London.

Pearson P and Spencer J (Eds) 1997 *Promoting Teamwork in Primary Care. A Research Based Approach.* Arnold, London.

UKCC 1992 *Scope of Professional Practice.* UKCC, London.

Unsworth J 2001 Developing primary care: the influence of society, policy and the professions. In: Spencer S, Unsworth J and Burke W (Eds) *Developing Community Nursing Practice.* Open University Press, Buckingham, pp. 11–36.

Wanless, D 2002 *Securing Our Future Health: Taking a Long-term View.* HM Treasury, London.

Watson NA and Wilkinson C (Eds) 2001 *Nursing in Primary Care. A Handbook for Students.* Palgrave, Basingstoke.

World Health Organization 1999 *Health21 – Health for All in the 21st Century. The Health for All Policy Framework for the WHO European Region.* World Health Organization Regional Office for Europe, Copenhagen.

NOTES

Note 1

Throughout this book we have used the terms Primary Care Groups and Primary Care Trusts (PCGs and PCTs) as the terms to refer to all the new primary-care organizations in the four countries of the United Kingdom, rather than having to repeat the titles of the bodies in each country each time while acknowledging the different structures and purposes of the different organizations in Northern Ireland, Scotland and Wales. We hope our colleagues in the other countries will be tolerant of this.

Note 2

The research assessment exercise is a review of research published by staff in university departments. It takes place every 4–5 years and is undertaken by the university funding system. The quality of the research is graded, providing a grade for each academic department. Research funding is then provided to departments according to the grade they achieved.

Section 1

2

Practice development: Defining the terms

Jane Griffiths

Purpose of this chapter

- To analyse definitions of practice development, research and implementation.
- To define what we mean by practice development in community nursing.
- To discuss the state of the art of practice development in community nursing.
- To describe the various terms commonly used in practice development.

INTRODUCTION

The terms that require clarification when discussing practice development in community nursing are many and varied. Before presenting examples of practice development in community nursing in subsequent chapters of this book, it is essential that a shared meaning of the terms that are in common use be provided. This chapter will start by discussing the term 'practice development' itself, to arrive at a definition that encompasses the range of activities community nurses are engaged in to improve their practice. It will then move on to an analysis of some of the other terms that come under, or are associated with, practice development.

WHAT IS PRACTICE DEVELOPMENT?

The definition of practice itself is non-contentious. Although there may be a lack of clarity at times about what various professions should be doing within community nursing, there is shared understanding of the broad term 'practice'. However, the meaning of development is far less clear. There appear to be significant contradictions in what is meant by it, with the activities that constitute 'development' variously defined throughout the NHS. These variations seem, on the whole, to concern the extent to which development is viewed as a rigorous process that should be subjected to the same scrutiny as empirical research. So, for example, while many people view development as a relatively slow process of trial and error that continues over a long period of time, for others it may be a short-term project that tests out a piece of research evidence in the field.

Development is one half of the NHS Research and Development strategy (Department of Health, 1993), and as such is actually fairly narrowly defined, as Russell (1996:4) explains:

> Development is the *experimental* introduction into practice of alternative clinical procedures or methods of care, together with the *simultaneous evaluation* of their effectiveness, efficiency or both. This includes health technology assessment, Phase III drug trials, and other pragmatic trials designed to choose between alternatives in clinical practice. It excludes service developments that are not subject to evaluation. [*my emphases*]

This definition has its roots in industry where a product is researched, produced and then tested out. The testing out is the 'development' component of the process that leads to refinement of the product before it is launched on to the market. According to this definition, therefore, development is more accurately described as applied research using, often, rigorous quantitative methods such as clinical trials.

Research is equally narrowly defined (Russell, 1996:4) as:

> ... scientific activity to test hypotheses and thus to generate new knowledge that may subsequently be useful in improving the effectiveness or efficiency of health care. This includes basic biomedical, psychological and sociological research, Phase I and Phase II drug trials, and other explanatory or fastidious trials designed to test scientific hypotheses.

The implication of this definition is that research studies that test hypotheses are the most relevant and applicable to improving health service efficiency and effectiveness. This excludes research that uses qualitative methods where rich description of phenomena in the context in which they occur is the aim, in other words, much of community nursing research.

It is useful to look at a similarly narrow definition of implementation before considering how these definitions may be broadened to describe practice development in community nursing (Russell, 1996:4):

> Implementation is the establishment in routine practice of clinical procedures or methods of care for which there is evidence of effectiveness and efficiency. This evidence should be derived from research or development or both, preferably through a systematic literature review.

This definition of implementation is probably closest to what most nurses understand by 'development' in clinical practice. An example is the application in practice of the Royal College of Nursing (RCN) clinical guidelines for the management of venous leg ulceration (Royal College of Nursing Institute, 1998), and the various measures taken to enable them to be adhered to, such as local protocols, leg ulcer clinics and the appointment of specialist nurses. Russell's narrow definition of implementation not only belies the complexity of implementing research in practice, but again requires evidence to be of a narrowly defined type. Systematic reviews define research evidence very rigidly, as that which is derived from randomized controlled trials.

It is important to consider these restrictive definitions of research, development and implementation because the quest for hard scientific evidence is the prevailing culture in much of the health service. If taken too literally, this drive for 'hard' evidence and 'experimental' application of that evidence in practice could stifle the creativity of practitioners engaging in important service developments. Developing practice is about more than implementing research findings. For community nurses, for example, reflection and critical thinking are also important activities that will lead to changes in practice.

For community nurses, narrow definitions of development are unhelpful, for the following reasons. There is little research evidence to draw on in many areas of community nursing practice and much of our research evidence comes from small-scale descriptive studies. We are a much 'newer' discipline than medicine in this respect and should not be dissuaded from developing our practice by a lack of research evidence. In any case, some of the evidence that we use to inform our practice may, through choice, always derive from small-scale qualitative studies, as much of our work is not amenable to measurement using other methods. Some developments may not be based on research findings at all (where such evidence is not available) but will still be conducted rigorously and systematically and may actually generate research questions.

A broader definition of development that encompasses the many activities community nurses are involved in to improve their practice comes from the National Health Service Executive (NHSE) publication *Achieving Effective Practice* (National Health Service Executive, 1998:6): 'Development [is] work directed towards introducing an innovation or the improvement of a service or process, often based on the findings of research'.

An *Effective Health Care* bulletin (NHS Centre for Reviews and Dissemination, 1999:2), which addressed methods for getting evidence into practice, considered many possible strategies:

> . . . research evidence from empirical studies of behaviour change; theoretical
> evidence from models of behavioural change derived from psychology, marketing and
> health promotion; and insights from case studies which have attempted to change
> professional practice within the NHS.

The method for developing practice is broadly defined therefore, and not restricted to the application in practice of research methods. Also, the innovation itself *may* be the application of a research finding, or it may not. What is missing from the NHSE (1998) definition, however, is the need for evaluation of developments in practice. Like Russell (1996), I would argue that evaluation of an innovation is essential. How else can success or otherwise of an intervention be determined, and changes to the process of implementation be made? A description of research is not given in the above document (National Health Service Executive, 1998), but the NHSE adapted a community nurse's definition of research (most recently updated in Hockey, 2000) in their glossary of terms: 'a systematic investigation undertaken to discover facts or relationships and reach conclusions using scientifically sound methods' (NHSE, 1998:6).

This broad description of the type of research that should be applied in practice is more realistic and relevant for community nurses, and less likely to stifle innovation than some of the other more restrictive definitions.

In this brief discussion of practice development, terms have already been used that may be unfamiliar to some readers. The remainder of this chapter explores terms relevant to practice development that are in common use in discussions about care of people in the community.

CLINICAL EFFECTIVENESS

In the past, community nursing has been based, to a large extent, on trial and error, personal experience and tradition. If a procedure worked, we were often unclear about why it worked, and if it did not work, we may either have been unaware of this, or may not have known how to find the best possible evidence for it. The aim of clinical effectiveness in practice is to change this haphazard way of deciding how to manage patient care to an approach that is overtly more systematic, economical, safe and knowledgeable. Put simply, clinical effectiveness is about doing the right thing in the right way at the right time for the right patient (Royal College of Nursing, 1996). Ideally this is based on evidence. So what is the difference, if any, between evidence-based practice and clinically effective practice?

There is much debate about what can be considered to be 'evidence' on which to base decisions about health care. In Chapter 3 of this book, José Closs argues for a narrow definition of evidence as that which is derived from rigorous research studies. She considers that, whereas other forms of knowledge, such as professional judgement, are important and used by community nurses in their decision making, they should not be regarded as evidence. Closs does, however, argue that clinically effective practice is only achievable where there is evidence for practice, clinical expertise, patient preference and the resources to implement care (see Fig. 3.1). Box 2.1 presents seven steps to such clinically effective practice. Although one of the steps involves searching for research to inform practice, it is also recognized that decisions may be based upon other types of information, such as expert opinion, discussion with colleagues and local audit.

It is accepted in the scientific community that there is a hierarchy of evidence, graded according to weight, with systematic reviews and randomized controlled trials at the top of the hierarchy and descriptive studies towards the bottom (see Table 3.2). Qualitative researchers would challenge this devaluing of their contribution to evidence-based practice, arguing that the findings of a well-conducted, in-depth qualitative study can be transferred usefully to other settings. Expert opinion as a form of evidence comes lower still in the hierarchy of evidence, occupying bottom position. Closs, in Chapter 3, argues that expert opinion as a form of evidence should not be relied upon, while other authors (Closs cites Le May, 1999) recommend using less rigorous evidence in the absence of anything stronger. It has already been discussed in this chapter that much of the activity of community nurses does not have a research base to underpin it. Where we do not know what clinically effective practice is, the NHSE (1998:6) recommends that:

Box 2.1 Seven steps to clinically effective practice

1. Are you certain that you are practising in a way that is clinically effective for the patients, i.e. the right way, which achieves the right results?
2. Do you know if any research studies have been done to examine different ways and determine which ways are best?
3. Are there any clinical guidelines available, which describe good practice based on research findings and/or expert opinion?
4. Have you and your colleagues discussed and agreed on good practice?
5. Have you and your colleagues carried out a clinical audit to confirm that you are following good practice on a day-to-day basis?
6. Have you acted to improve your practice if needed?
7. Have you shared your experiences in implementing good practice with other nurses?

(National Health Service Executive, 1998:6)

It's best to see what respected experts in the area of practice recommend as best practice. If experts haven't yet considered what best practice is for a particular area of care, the next best action is to seek advice from national, regional or local resource centres or individuals or to reach consensus with your colleagues on what you think best practice should be locally.

The majority of exponents of evidence-based practice would hesitate before calling this type of information evidence, yet for a substantial amount of community nursing practice, if developments are to occur, this is the best knowledge currently available.

So, at one end of the spectrum of evidence is expert or consensus opinion, and at the other is research, using what are often considered to be the most rigorous scientific methods, the randomized controlled trial and the systematic review.

RANDOMIZED CONTROLLED TRIALS

At the opposite end of the spectrum of evidence from expert or consensus opinion is the randomized controlled trial. As a well-designed randomized controlled trial (RCT) is often considered to be the best form of evidence, it is important to explain what is meant by this research design (Shepperd *et al.*, 1997).

An RCT is a clinical trial in which the patients are randomly allocated to a group receiving an intervention, such as a drug, or to a control group that will not be receiving the intervention, but may be receiving a placebo. The groups are matched as far as possible so that it is the effect of the intervention that is being observed rather than some extraneous variable. The groups are, in theory, otherwise identical. In the development of a new drug, a series of RCTs are conducted, termed Phase I, II, III and IV studies, in increasingly more general populations (*see* Chapter 6).

Although often viewed as the best form of evidence when seeking out research to support practice, RCTs are only useful when answering certain research questions. They are useful for comparing drugs, surgical interventions or, possibly, health education interventions. They would be inappropriate, for example, where the quality of care was being studied rather than the success of a surgical intervention (Greenhalgh, 2001). There are also occasions where it would be unethical to randomize patients into an intervention or control group, such as when it is highly likely that the intervention is more beneficial or harmful than the control, or where patients express a clear preference (*see* Chapter 8).

As with all research, it is important to use the right design to answer the question posed, rather than using a research design simply because it is valued more highly by the academic community.

SYSTEMATIC REVIEWS

A systematic review of the literature can be considered to be research in itself. The aim is to summarize an otherwise unwieldy body of research evidence for the reader by looking at all of the research literature available to answer a question, and drawing comparisons. Drawing comparisons between research studies can either be carried out statistically using a method called meta-analysis (*see* below) or qualitatively by developing common themes. Good examples of high-quality and clearly written systematic reviews are found in the widely available *Effective Health Care* bulletins published by the Centre for Reviews and Dissemination in York, many of which are relevant to community nurses, such as venous leg ulcer management and breastfeeding. The Centre for Reviews and Dissemination is funded by the government to conduct systematic reviews and distribute them to health service personnel. Another source of systematic reviews is the increasingly comprehensive Cochrane database of systematic reviews, which these days should probably be your first port of call when searching for evidence on a topic. Information on both of these sources of information can be found in Chapter 12 of this book.

In the first instance, the researcher carrying out a systematic review will look for RCTs conducted in the field. The RCT is considered to be the best form of evidence to establish the *effectiveness* of a certain type of treatment, and it is often the effectiveness of something that a systematic review is trying to establish. In some circumstances RCTs will not have been conducted or are not the most appropriate research design to answer the question, so other research designs are included in the review.

Details of how to carry out a systematic review are available (*see*, for example, NHS Centre for Reviews and Dissemination, 1996). It is by no means a simple process, but to summarize, the process basically involves seven steps (Box 2.2).

Well-conducted systematic reviews are an invaluable resource for community nurses. One piece of research evidence may give a very unbalanced picture of best practice. A summary of a body of literature is a far more reliable source of evidence. If the review is from a reliable source, a skilled researcher or team of researchers will have critiqued the quality of the individual pieces of research, which can save valu-

---

Box 2.2 Seven steps to carrying out a systematic review

1. Arrive at a well-defined question for the review, which includes the target population, health care intervention and outcomes of interest.
2. Decide which studies should be included or excluded, and on what grounds.
3. Systematically collect all of the available literature on the topic, using, for example, electronic databases, hand-searching journals, and seeking out the grey (unpublished) literature.
4. Assess the literature for inclusion in the review by applying the inclusion and exclusion criteria from step two.
5. Assess the quality or validity of the included studies.
6. Extract relevant information from the selected studies.
7. Synthesize the information using either qualitative or quantitative methods (meta-analysis).

---

able time. Not all systematic reviews are conducted rigorously, however, and while reviews from the Cochrane or Campbell Collaboration or the NHS Centre for Reviews and Dissemination for example, are likely to be reliable, community nurses need to know how to evaluate the quality of systematic reviews (*see*, for example, Greenhalgh, 2001).

META-ANALYSIS

When a number of studies on the same topic are looked at, some of them may have statistically significant findings and others might not. A classic example of this is found in seven trials of the effect of giving steroids to mothers who had a high chance of giving birth prematurely, and therefore of having babies with immature lungs and associated breathing difficulties. However, only two of the seven clinical trials demonstrated a statistically significant benefit of administering steroids in terms of survival of the infant. In the other five trials there was an observable benefit that was of clinical significance but it was not statistically significant. When further statistical analysis was applied to the pooled results of all seven studies, however, the result was in favour of administering steroids to mothers who were at risk of going into labour prematurely (*see* Greenhalgh, 2001, Chapter 12 for a more extensive discussion of this evidence). This technique of secondary analysis is called *meta-analysis*. Greenhalgh (2001:129) defines meta-analysis as: 'a statistical synthesis of the numerical results of several trials which all addressed the same question'.

Readers may be familiar with the logo of the Cochrane Collaboration (Fig. 2.1). This is a visual representation of the meta-analysis described above. Put very simply, the seven horizontal lines correspond to the seven clinical trials. The vertical line is the 'line of no effect'. If the horizontal line representing the trial does not cross the vertical line there is a 95% chance that there is a real difference between the experimental group and the control group in the trial; in this case, that the use of steroids

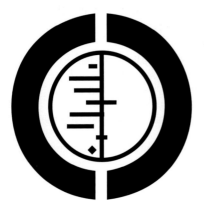

Fig. 2.1 *The logo of the Cochrane Collaboration (reproduced with permission from the Cochrane Collaboration).*

increased the survival of pre-term infants. The diamond represents the pooled results of the seven trials. The fact that it is narrower in width than the individual lines demonstrates that the strength of the evidence is in favour of administering steroids to pre-term infants. A fuller, rather more complex, but very readable, account of meta-analysis can be found in *How to Read a Paper* by Greenhalgh (2001).

CRITICAL APPRAISAL SKILLS

If a systematic review has not been carried out on the topic about which you are interested, it is necessary to critically appraise the individual study or studies that you have found. In this context, critical appraisal means looking at the different sections of a paper, starting with the question and method, to establish whether there are important flaws in the study. Critical appraisal skills are not straightforward and cannot be acquired overnight. If there is an opportunity to attend a critical appraisal skills workshop or course in your place of work, this is an excellent way to begin to develop the skills required. Individuals or groups could also undertake the self-study workbook written by Greenhalgh and Donald (2000). It is important to remember, however, that some of the skills needed when making an initial assessment of the quality of a paper require straightforward common sense, something which community nurses have plenty of! Based on your knowledge of the subject area and the people being studied, is what the researchers have done sensible, or are there some obvious problems with the research?

For examples of the more obvious flaws to be found in research papers, you are directed again to Greenhalgh's excellent, accessible text *How to Read a Paper* (Greenhalgh, 2001). When looking at a clinical trial or survey, for example, she suggests that it is important to ask whether the patients differed in important ways from the 'average' patient. In order to test the intervention, did they have no other health problem apart from the condition being researched? Were they more ill or less ill than real-life patients? Did they receive the type of attention throughout the study that real-life patients could not possibly receive? Was their lifestyle, their ethnic background, or habits such as smoking and alcohol consumption the same as that of the average patient?

As far as the statistical section of quantitative papers is concerned, Greenhalgh (2001:69) suggests rather reassuringly (to the less mathematically inclined among us!) that:

> As a non-statistician, I tend to look for three numbers in the methods section of a paper:
>
> 1. the size of the sample
> 2. the duration of follow-up
> 3. the completeness of follow-up.

Her book is full of commonsensical advice about how to read critically without becoming baffled.

Similar advice can be offered when reading qualitative papers. For example, when looking at the methods section of a qualitative paper, it is the level of detail that explains the 'decision-making trial' of the researcher that is crucial. All too often qualitative papers reach fascinating conclusions without making it absolutely clear how they were arrived at. The sample should be one that is capable of offering the maximum insight into a phenomenon – a biased sample, in other words – and rarely, if ever, one of convenience.

Fear of reading research papers – quantitative papers in particular – should not lead nurses to believe that if it is published and it is 'research', then it must be true. A common sense approach to reading research will reveal a lot about the quality of the work before you start deciding whether the statistical test used was appropriate or not.

CLINICAL GUIDELINES

National clinical guidelines that have been endorsed by professional organizations, commended by the NHSE, and latterly the National Institute for Clinical Excellence (NICE), who also commission guidelines (see below), are increasingly available to community nurses to inform their practice. Clinical guidelines have been defined as: ' . . . systematically developed statements to assist practitioners' decisions about appropriate health care for specific clinical circumstances' (Field and Lohr, 1990, cited by Greenhalgh, 2001:140). Protocols and care pathways are more prescriptive in their guidance and therefore more restrictive, i.e. they tell the practitioner what should be done and (often) when. Guidelines allow practitioners to use more of their own clinical judgement and discretion in implementing them. This does not mean that guidelines can be disregarded, but that they offer evidence-based guidance (Hurwitz, 1998).

Before developing guidelines from scratch locally, it is sensible to see whether any guidelines have been produced nationally that can be adapted to suit local need. National guidelines that have been approved by the NHSE or NICE will invariably have been developed over a longer period of time and with greater access to clinical expertise than is available to individuals locally.

Ideally, the guidelines are based on systematic reviews of the available research, as it is this type of evidence that is most reliable. Guidelines take systematic reviews one step further by offering guidance on how the evidence can be applied in practice. Examples of national clinical guidelines that are relevant to community nurses are: the management of patients with venous leg ulcers (Royal College of Nursing Institute, 1998; *see* Box 2.3) and pressure ulcer risk assessment and prevention (Rycroft-Malone and Duff, 2000).

Box 2.3 Excerpt from *The Management of Venous Leg Ulcers* (Royal College of Nursing Institute, 1998)

Pain assessment and relief

2.3 Health professionals should regularly monitor whether patients experience pain associated with venous leg ulcers and formulate an individual management plan, which may consist of compression therapy, exercise, leg elevation and analgesia, to meet the needs of the patient.

Rationale

A significant proportion of patients with venous ulcers report moderate to severe pain (Hamer *et al.*, 1994; Cullum and Roe, 1995; Walshe, 1995; Dunn *et al.*, 1997; Hofman *et al.*, 1997, Stevens *et al.*, 1997). Yet one survey found that 55 per cent of district nurses did not assess patient's pain (Roe *et al.*, 1993). Increased pain on mobility may be associated with poorer healing rates (Johnson, 1995) and may also be a sign of some underlying pathology such as arterial disease or infection (indicating that the patient requires referral for some specialized assessment).

Leg elevation is important since it can aid venous return and reduce pain and swelling in some patients. However, leg elevation may make the pain worse in others (Hofman *et al.*, 1997). Compression counteracts the harmful effects of venous hypertension and compression may relieve pain (Franks *et al.*, 1992). Exercise maintains the venous calf pump function.

Fifty per cent of patients with purely venous aetiology reporting severe pain are taking either mild analgesia or none at all (Hofman *et al.*, 1997). Analgesics containing opioids may be necessary in some patients.

Strength of evidence (II)

Although the research is quite heterogeneous, the results consistently report that patients with venous leg ulcers can experience considerable pain (one prospective, one matched and two cross-sectional studies). There is also some evidence that pain relief occurs with compression and healing (Franks *et al.*, 1992). No research could be identified that examined the use of a pain assessment method specifically designed for patients with venous leg ulcers, or that compared different forms of relief. There is very little conclusive research on other pain relief strategies such as exercise and leg elevation.

References

Cullum N and Roe B 1995 *Leg ulcers. Nursing management – a research based guide.* Baillière Tindall, London.

Dunn C, Beegan A and Morris S (1997) Towards evidence based practice. *Focus on venous ulcers.* Mid term review progress report compiled for King's Fund PACE project. King's Fund, London.

Franks PJ, Wright DDI, Fletcher AE *et al.* (1992) A questionnaire to assess risk factors, quality of life and use of health resources in patients with venous disease. *European Journal of Surgery* 158: 149–55.

Hamer C, Cullum NA and Roe BH (1994) Patient's perceptions of chronic leg ulcers. *Journal of Wound Care* 3(2): 99–102.

Hofman D, Ryan TJ, Arnold F *et al.* (1997) Pain in venous leg ulcers. *Journal of Wound Care* 6(5): 222–4.

Johnson M 1995 Patient characteristics and environmental factors in leg ulcer healing. *Journal of Wound Care* 4(6): 277–82.

Roe BH, Luker KA, Cullum NA *et al.* 1993 Assessment prevention and monitoring of chronic leg ulcers in the community: report of a survey. *Journal of Clinical Nursing* 2: 299–306.

Stevens J, Franks PJ and Harrington M 1997 A community/hospital leg ulcer service. *Journal of Wound Care* 6(2): 62–8.

Walshe C (1995) Living with a venous ulcer: a descriptive study of patients' experiences. *Journal of Advanced Nursing* 22(6): 92–100.

The simple introduction of clinical guidelines does seem to lead to changes in practice. However, in a systematic review of the effectiveness of implementing clinical practice guidelines (University of Leeds, 1994), when summarizing the evidence the reviewers concluded that the introduction of guidelines *can* change clinical practice and affect patient outcome, but that the way that guidelines are developed, implemented and monitored seems to influence uptake. They also noted that guidelines are likely to be more effective if they take into account local circumstances and are disseminated by an active educational intervention (*see* Chapters 6 and 7 in this volume).

NATIONAL INSTITUTE FOR CLINICAL EXCELLENCE

The National Institute for Clinical Excellence (NICE) is a Special Health Authority that was set up in April 1999 as part of the government's quality improvement agenda. The aim of NICE is to eradicate current inconsistencies in clinical standards across the country by introducing guidance, guidelines and audit. To achieve this, the approach presented in Box 2.4 has been implemented (Department of Health, 1998).

NICE aims to operate as a single, central body through which existing and new guidelines for practice will be assessed and disseminated. The guidelines programme contains several topics that are relevant to community nurses, such as the treatment and prevention of pressure sores, depressive illness in the community and the management of completed myocardial infarction in primary care. The guidance produced by NICE is not mandatory, but the Commission for Health Improvement (CHI) will be assessing how the guidance and guidelines have been adopted locally,

---

Box 2.4 Purpose of the National Institute for Clinical Excellence

1. Identification:
   - Of new health interventions that will have a significant impact on the health service
   - Of existing interventions where there are variations in practice or uncertainties about clinical and cost effectiveness
2. Collecting evidence: carrying out research to establish the clinical and cost effectiveness of interventions
3. Appraisal and guidance: appraising the evidence on clinical and cost effectiveness and producing guidelines for practitioners
4. Dissemination of guidelines and audit tools for monitoring uptake
5. Implementation of guidelines locally
6. Monitoring the process and constantly updating information as new research emerges, taking into account patient views.

(Department of Health, 1998)

---

and may ask for demonstration of this. As well as troubleshooting, CHI offers support to those organizations that fall below national standards.

Although the government has made it very clear that the guidance offered is to be developed in an inclusive fashion, and implemented in partnership with local organizations, NICE is essentially a centrally led, 'top-down' approach to developing practice. This is not to suggest that the initiative is inappropriate as, clearly, variations in clinical services across the country are unacceptable, but that it is just one of a spectrum of approaches that are currently available for raising clinical standards.

Also the guidelines are at present clinically focused. Although guidelines that are applicable to the primary health care setting are important for community nurses working in multidisciplinary teams, they may be of greater relevance to community nursing disciplines with a stronger clinical component to their work.

NATIONAL SERVICE FRAMEWORKS

National Service Frameworks (NSFs) are evidence-based standards that are being developed for major care areas and disease groups. They are defined as:

> . . . key new tools tackling major health issues and important diseases. Their purpose is to improve health, reduce inequalities and raise the quality of care . . . NSFs set out both the vision for the future and the practical short and medium term actions required to achieve that vision.

(Department of Health, 2000a:5)

The Calman–Hine report prototype NSF for cancer services (Department of Health, 2000b) and the NSFs for Coronary Heart Disease, Mental Health and Older

> **Box 2.5 Purpose of a National Service Framework**
>
> - A description of the scope of the NSF
> - The evidence base, including a needs assessment, evidence of clinical and cost effectiveness and present performance
> - National standards with timescales for delivery
> - Key interventions and costings
> - Commissioned work to support the implementation of the NSF, such as research and development (NHS R&D), benchmarking, outcome indicators
> - Supporting programmes, such as education and training, workforce planning, development activities (personal and organisational)
> - A performance management framework.
>
> (Department of Health, 1998)

People are early examples. NSFs contain an implementation and monitoring strategy. Box 2.5 shows what each NSF will comprise.

Again, to implement NSFs, the emphasis is on partnership with a wide range of organizations, both nationally and locally, to include social service providers, the voluntary sector and other government departments. It is clear that National Service Frameworks is an initiative that is of great relevance to community nurses, and it is important that you are involved in programmes of implementation of NSFs at all levels within your organization.

CLINICAL GOVERNANCE

Clinical governance is, quite simply, the umbrella term that is used to describe how all of the initiatives described so far are put into practice locally by organizations. It is essentially about ensuring quality improvement, and the responsibility of the organization to put systems in place to ensure that these improvements happen. The approaches being adopted are many and varied, and determined by local need. The government (Department of Health, 1998:33) defined it thus:

> Clinical governance can be defined as a framework through which NHS organisations are accountable for continuously improving the quality of their services and safeguarding high standards of care by creating an environment in which excellence in care standards will flourish.

The introduction of clinical governance to NHS organizations involves, most importantly, a change in culture. The theory is that organizations will be able to move away from a blame culture to one of *learning* through mistakes; and that staff at all levels will be involved in initiatives to improve the quality of services, breaking down inflexible professional barriers in the process (National Health Service Executive, 1999; Hittinger, 2002). The theoretical underpinnings are highly commendable;

success is likely to rely heavily on the management of individual organizations, in particular Primary Care Trusts.

For a digestible text containing suggestions on how to implement clinical governance, *see* Lugon and Secker-Walker (1999) *Clinical governance: making it happen.*

AUDIT

Audit monies are widely available for organizations to develop projects to assess whether quality improvements have taken place. Importantly, from your point of view, resources are available for community nurses to carry out projects to monitor standards in practice. For some time, audit has been an excellent way, perhaps the only way, of securing money and protected time for project work.

Audit has received a bad press in the past, and probably deservedly. Characteristically, audits were carried out by a person from outside the discipline being audited, as a one-off project that highlighted problems. This was written up in a report which, rather than being acted upon, sat on a shelf somewhere, gathering dust. Soul destroying for practitioners and a waste of resources!

The only way to conduct audit is as part of the audit cycle (Fig. 2.2). Audits should be carried out as many times as it takes to demonstrate that the standards set are being met. The basic aim of an audit is to set evidence-based standards; to devise a method to find out whether the standards are being reached, i.e. by measuring existing practice against best practice; *to develop practice* to help practitioners to meet standards they are currently not meeting; and then to re-audit, and so the cycle

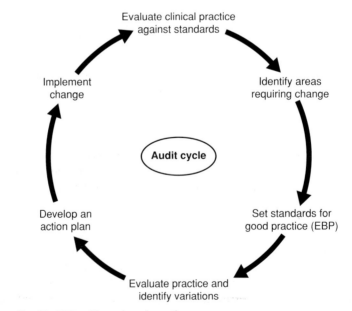

Fig. 2.2 *Audit cycle. EBP, evidence-based practice.*

continues (*see* Joyce Marshall's example of this in Chapter 6). There is a renewed emphasis on the value of audit to develop practice within the context of organizations that are committed to clinical governance (National Institute for Clinical Excellence, 2002).

Community nurses should be leading audit projects, where appropriate, although in my experience this is quite rare. Audits should also, in many cases, be multidisciplinary, because the quality of a service is rarely dependent on one discipline. It is important for you as community nurses to contact your audit department, find out how to apply for funding (often by a very straightforward proposal) and to become involved in this work if it interests you. In this way, you can release time for yourselves to become involved in practice development and, if the audit is nurse-led and conducted as a cycle rather than linearly, it should give you considerable scope for making quality improvements locally.

CRITICAL THINKING

Critical thinking is central to everything that has been discussed in this chapter and, indeed, in this book. By the same token, every chapter that you read in the book, including this, should be read critically! Readers who have recently embarked on Level 3 studies will be aware that the most important element of both your academic work and your clinical practice is the ability to think critically.

Critical thinking is different from other forms of thinking, such as creative thinking or the automatic thinking that we employ when carrying out repetitive tasks. Brookfield (1993) describes the characteristics of critical ability as reflective scepticism, identifying and challenging assumptions, and imagining and exploring alternatives. Critical thinking is not therefore a passive state. It requires the nurse to interact with the information received. Often, the critical thinker will not arrive at a solution, merely a series of questions, or ideas to be tested. Being critical is about living with uncertainty, and rarely with fact.

Critical thinking is important because nothing should be taken at face value. Just because something has always been done a certain way or because a certain belief has always shaped our practice, it does not mean that this should not be challenged. The physical isolation of community nurses in people's homes can mean that a lot of practice is never overseen. There is considerable scope for nurses to develop individualized approaches to their work based on habit rather than a sound rationale.

To take some examples from community nursing practice, consider the assumptions that are presented in Box 2.6. Do you or any of your colleagues hold these beliefs and, if so, what are the alternative ways of viewing each of these statements? What evidence, from either research or reflection on practice, supports these assumptions? Is there evidence from similar sources to refute them?

Critical thinking is about challenging practice and constantly asking 'why?', 'how?', 'what evidence do I have?', 'is there a better way of doing this?'. Critical thinking is therefore an essential activity in the process of clinical supervision (*see* Chapter 7). In the absence of quality research evidence, critical thinking and reflection, combined with personal expertise, may be the best knowledge base available to you.

Box 2.6 Assumptions to be challenged in primary health care

1. It is not possible to carry out health education/health promotion with older people.
2. Patients/clients often do not want to be empowered to make decisions about their health care.
3. Some patients/clients are non-compliant with treatment/management regimes.
4. If something is in print, it is true.
5. Nurses should not challenge the practice of another nursing colleague of the same grade.
6. It is important not to set a precedent when caring for a patient/client, because it is not possible to change the care at a later date.

REFLECTION

Reflection on practice is a means of appraising what has happened in the past, so that changes can be made to improve patient care. Critical thinking skills are needed to reflect on clinical practice, but, equally, it is claimed that the formal process of reflection can help nurses to develop their critical ability (Schon, 1983). Reflection or 'reflection-on-experience' is defined by Johns (1998:1) as:

> . . . a window for practitioners to look inside and know who they are as they strive towards understanding and realising the meaning of desirable work in their everyday practices. The practitioner must expose, confront and understand the contradictions within their practice, between what is practised and what is desirable. It is the conflict of contradiction and the commitment to achieve desirable work that empowers the practitioner to take action to appropriately resolve these contradictions.

Benner's interpretation (Benner, 1984) is that the novice practitioner breaks down care into its various components, but that the expert practitioner intuitively responds to the whole situation. This she describes as 'tacit knowing'. It is 'tacit' because if the expert practitioner is asked to reflect on the components of an episode of care afterwards, she may have considerable difficulty doing so. Not surprisingly, intuition is not the sort of knowledge that is readily accepted in the current climate of evidence-based practice, yet Benner contends that it is 'an unknowable' process. Other authors (Johns, 1998; Rolfe, 1998) would argue that there is 'knowable' logic in the process of clinical judgement, and that structured reflection can help the practitioner to articulate this knowledge, and make best use of it. Johns considers that reflection should always be guided if it is to serve its purpose of elucidating and articulating tacit past events. He proposes a model of structured reflection, shown in Box 2.7.

When we talk about reflection in nursing, we are invariably referring to the critical appraisal of past experiences. This type of reflection *after the event* is described by Schon as reflection-on-action. Schon does, however, describe another type of reflection, which he defines as reflection-in-action. This occurs *during* an event and changes the course of action that the nurse takes. Rolfe points out that this important form of reflection is entirely at odds with Benner's notion of intuition, where the

Box 2.7 A model of structured reflection

Write a description of the experience.
What are the specific issues I need to pay attention to?
Reflective cues:

- Aesthetics
  What was I trying to achieve?
  Why did I respond as I did?
  What were the consequences of that for:
      The patient?
      Others?
      Myself?
  How was this person feeling?
  How did I know this?
- Personal
  How did I feel in this situation?
  What internal factors were influencing me?
- Ethics
  How did my actions match with my beliefs?
  What factors made me act in incongruent ways?
- Empirics
  What knowledge did or should have informed me?
- Reflexivity
  How does this connect with previous experiences?
  Could I handle this better in similar situations?
  What would be the consequences be of alternative actions for:
      The patient?
      Others?
      Myself?
  How do I *now* feel about this experience?
  Can I support myself and others better as a consequence?
  Has this changed my ways of knowing?

(Johns, 1998:6)

expert practitioner, by definition, would not attend to the minutiae of the decision-making process.

Rolfe and Schon argue that *evidence* for a nurse's actions can be produced through reflection-in-action. Knowledge is produced, a form of research, perhaps, if not the kind of research evidence that the Department of Health had in mind! Irrespective of this, the reflexive practitioner, unlike the 'expert', can justify his or her decisions using reasoned argument.

Critics and supporters of reflection point out that we do not, as yet, have any research evidence that reflection changes practice. Neither do we know whether the process of reflection develops critical ability in nurses (Burton, 2000), which is one of the claims made for it (by Schon [1983], for example). Perhaps, however, critical skills come first.

It makes 'intuitive' sense that if an event is reflected on critically after it has happened, possible processes for changing practice can then be developed and tested. However, intuitively knowing that reflection makes sense is no substitute for robust evaluation. The relationship between reflection and research appears to be threefold: reflection as a form of evidence where research evidence is lacking; reflection as a means of getting research evidence into practice; and reflection as a means of changing practice *per se*. All three should ideally be evaluated using research methods.

CONCLUSION

This discussion of reflection ends this analysis of terms that are commonly associated with practice development. The message that I have tried to convey in this chapter is that although in the ideal world community nursing practice may be based on hard scientific evidence tested out in the field using rigorous research methods, this is far from reality. We *do* have access to relevant high-quality evidence to inform our practice, but where we do not, this should not stifle our attempts to improve practice. The ability to think critically and to reflect on our practice is invaluable to us as community nurses. In some cases it may be the best evidence available.

Quality in the health service is valued by the present government. Community nurses are part of an organizational culture where numerous initiatives are in place to help us to develop our practice. It is essential that we seize the opportunities that have become available to us at all levels of the organizations in which we work.

REFERENCES

Benner P 1984 *From Novice to Expert*. Addison Wesley, Menlo Park.

Brookfield S 1993 On impostership, cultural suicide, and other dangers: how nurses learn critical thinking. *Journal of Continuing Education in Nursing* 24(5): 197–205.

Burton AJ 2000 Reflection: nursing's practice and education panacea? *Journal of Advanced Nursing* 31(5): 1009–17.

Department of Health 1993 *Research for Health*. HMSO, London.

Department of Health 1998 *A First Class Service: Quality in the New NHS*. HMSO, London.

Department of Health 2000a *National Service Framework: Coronary Heart Disease*. Modern Standards and Service Models. Department of Health, London.

Department of Health 2000b *NHS Cancer Plan*. Department of Health, London.

Field MJ and Lohr KN 1990 *Clinical Practice Guidelines: Direction of a New Agency*. Institute of Medicine, Washington DC.

Greenhalgh T 2001 *How to Read a Paper: The Basis of Evidence Based Medicine*, 2nd edition. BMJ Publishing Group, London.

Greenhalgh T and Donald A 2000 *Evidence Based Health Care Workbook. For individual and group learning*. BMJ Publishing Group, London.

Hittinger R 2002 Using clinical indicators to achieve clinical governance. *Clinical Governance Bulletin* 3(1): 4–5.

Hockey L 2000 The nature and purpose of research. Chapter 1 in: Cormack DFS (Ed.) 2000 *The Research Process in Nursing 4th Edn.* Blackwell Science, Oxford. Cited in NHSE (1998) National Health Service Executive 1999.

Hurwitz B 1998 *Clinical Guidelines and the Law.* Radcliffe Medical Press Ltd, Abingdon.

Johns C 1998 Opening the doors of perception. In: Johns C and Freshwater D (Eds) *Transforming Nursing Through Reflective Practice.* Blackwell Science, Oxford, pp. 1–20.

Le May A 1999 *Evidence-based Practice.* Nursing Times Clinical Monograph No. 1. NT Books, London.

Lugon M and Secker-Walker J 1999 *Clinical Governance: Making it Happen.* The Royal Society of Medicine Press Ltd, London.

NHS Centre for Reviews and Dissemination 1996 *CRD Guidelines for those Carrying Out or Commissioning Reviews.* CRD Report Number 4, January. University of York, York.

NHS Centre for Reviews and Dissemination 1999 Getting evidence into practice. *Effective Health Care* bulletin 5(1).

National Health Service Executive 1998 *Achieving Effective Practice: A Clinical Effectiveness and Research Information Pack for Nurses, Midwives and Health Visitors.* NHSE, Leeds.

National Health Service Executive 1999 *Clinical Governance.* NHSE, Leeds.

National Institute for Clinical Excellence 2002 *Principles for Best Practice in Clinical Audit.* Radcliffe Medical Press, Abingdon.

Rolfe G 1998 Beyond expertise: reflective and reflexive nursing practice. In: Johns C and Freshwater D (Eds) *Transforming Nursing Through Reflective Practice.* Blackwell Science, Oxford, pp. 21–31.

Royal College of Nursing 1996 *Clinical Effectiveness: a Royal College of Nursing guide.* RCN, London.

Royal College of Nursing Institute 1998 *Clinical Practice Guidelines for the Management of Patients with Venous Leg Ulcers: Recommendations for Assessment, Compression Therapy, Cleansing, Debridement, Dressings, Contact Sensitivity.* Royal College of Nursing and Centre for Evidence-Based Nursing, School of Nursing Midwifery and Health Visiting, University of Manchester. RCN Publishing, London.

Dunn II I 1990 What is research and development? *Refocus: The NHSE Northern and Yorkshire Research and Development Newsletter* Issue 4, Spring: 4–5.

Rycroft-Malone J and Duff L 2000 Pressure ulcer risk assessment and prevention: clinical practice guidelines. *Nursing Standard* 14(40): 31.

Schon DA 1983 *The Reflective Practitioner.* Avebury, Aldershot.

Shepperd S, Doll H and Jenkinson C 1997 Randomized controlled trials. In: Jenkinson C (Ed.) *Assessment and Evaluation of Health and Medical Care.* Open University Press, Buckingham, pp. 31–46.

University of Leeds 1994 Implementing clinical practice guidelines. *Effective Health Care* December, Number 8.

3

Evidence and community-based nursing practice

S. José Closs

Purpose of this chapter

- To examine the nature of evidence.
- To describe the characteristics of evidence-based nursing.
- To consider the quality of currently available evidence.
- To examine some of the issues concerned with evidence-based practice in community and primary-care nursing.

INTRODUCTION

The development of nursing practice depends on many things. A crucial factor is the availability and use of high-quality evidence in the development process. For nursing, this first became enshrined in policy in 1972, when the Briggs report recommended that the profession should be research based: 'Nursing should become a research-based profession' (Briggs, 1972:108). In 1993, the NHS Management Executive stated that: 'nursing research should be integrated into primary care nursing practice. Existing practice should be continuously evaluated to ensure that every nursing activity is demonstrably beneficial to individual patient outcome and population health gain' (NHS Management Executive, 1993:39). This sentiment was reiterated in the Mant report on research and development in primary care (NHS Executive, 1997).

When considering evidence-based nursing (EBN) there is a range of issues of concern to nurses based in the community, some theoretical and some practical. The theoretical issues are concerned with understanding what constitutes 'good' evidence – these are of general concern to all health care professionals. However, many of the practical issues involved in accessing, appraising and implementing evidence are very specific to particular situations encountered by community nurses (Bryar, 1999).

The phrase 'evidence-based nursing' rolls easily off the tongue, but in reality it is a complex activity. A considerable amount of skill is needed in order to track down and appraise evidence before deciding whether or not it would be appropriate to use it.

Then there is the not inconsiderable task of successfully introducing it into everyday practice, using methods such as those discussed in Chapter 4 and Section 2. The sceptics have described evidence-based health care (EBH) as a: ' . . . fashionable tendency . . . to belittle the performance of experienced clinicians by using a combination of epidemiological jargon and statistical sleight-of-hand' (Greenhalgh, 2001: 3). On the face of it this sounds damning, but statistics and at least some jargon are necessary parts of some research and they can be understood with some effort.

There is, however, an element of truth in the notion of fashion here; after all, for two or three decades nursing has been struggling to develop its research base in order to provide evidence-based care. Although terminology changes over time, many of the issues do not, and the push from the Department of Health for EBH simply extends the efforts the profession was already making. Indeed, the introduction of the ethos of evidence-based care across all health care professions should make our progress easier. EBN should emphatically not, however, belittle either experienced clinicians or the views of patients and carers, as discussed below.

EVIDENCE: WHAT IT IS AND WHAT IT ISN'T

The *Oxford English Dictionary* (1994) defines evidence as: 'ground for belief, testimony or facts tending to prove or disprove any conclusion'. Implicit in this definition are two key notions, namely that evidence must be convincing ('ground for *belief*'), and that evidence confirms or refutes a conclusion rather than producing absolute truth ('*tending* to prove or disprove'). Evidence may not provide certainty, but it should remove all reasonable doubt.

Evidence-based medicine has been defined as:

> The conscientious, explicit and judicious use of current best evidence in making decisions about the care of individual patients. The practice of evidence-based medicine means integrating individual clinical expertise with the best available external evidence from systematic research.
>
> (Sackett *et al.*, 1996:71)

This definition places emphasis on three elements: 'current best evidence', 'external evidence' and the integration of the evidence with individual clinical expertise.

The reference to 'current best evidence' indicates the constantly changing nature of evidence – as more research is completed over time, the picture of the phenomenon under study tends to become clearer, and may change, either subtly or dramatically. As research progresses, we get nearer to the 'truth' about a phenomenon, but it is unlikely that we can ever achieve absolute certainty. We therefore aim to give the best care we can, given the current availability of reliable evidence. This means that keeping up to date with research is important. For example, it had been routine 'best' practice in health visiting for many years to undertake a distraction-hearing test on all babies at the age of 6–9 months to identify hearing loss. In the Third Hall Report (Hall, 1996) the problems with this test were summarized from the available evidence:

- The sensitivity of the test is often low and cases are missed.

- Poor technique results in a large number of false positives.
- Coverage is often unsatisfactory.
- Hearing loss in non-attenders is higher than in attenders.
- Parental concerns and risk factors are often ignored.
- Many transient cases due to middle-ear infection are identified.

Evidence of the effectiveness of the health visitor distraction test (HVDT) and neonatal hearing screening (which uses technological measures) to detect infants with congenital hearing loss was reviewed by Davis *et al.* (1997). The main conclusions, shown in Box 3.1, indicate that current best practice to detect congenital hearing loss requires the provision of a neonatal hearing screening service enabling detection at a much earlier age.

These conclusions indicate that current and ongoing research demonstrate the greater superiority of neonatal hearing screening. However, the translation of such findings into everyday practice is not without problems. Although the introduction of a national neonatal hearing screening service would prevent distress to parents and children missed by the distraction test, and would also free up the time of health visitors and others involved in the HVDT to enable them to spend their time more effectively, the actual adoption of neonatal testing has to take into account: competing health service priorities; professional vested interest; parental views; logistical difficulties to ensure coverage and many other factors affecting the process of changing practice (*see* Chapter 4). This massive change in the organization of services is being managed by an implementation team from the Medical Research Council Institute of Hearing Research. Twenty pilot sites for implementation have been chosen and lessons from the evaluation of the implementation in these sites will inform the implementation throughout the country (Hind *et al.*, 2001).

Sackett's definition identifies 'external evidence' as the second most important criterion. Convincing evidence must be in the public realm, that is, it must be available to anyone who wishes to consider it. The process by which the evidence was produced must be clearly stated, so that it can be subjected to proper scrutiny and its

---

Box 3.1 Evidence indicating a need to reconsider 'best' practice in detecting congenital hearing loss

- 'There are approximately 840 children a year born in the UK with a significant permanent hearing impairment . . . Present services will miss about 400 of these children by 1½ years of age, and about 200 of these children by 3½ years of age.'
- 'The published evidence on screening performance indicates poor sensitivity and relatively poor specificity for the HVDT, with relatively low yield. Median age of identification via the HVDT varies from 12 to 20 months.
- 'Neonatal screening shows high test sensitivity and reasonably high programme sensitivity, with high specificity. The limited number of universal neonatal screening programmes implemented at present give yields of the expected order.'
- 'Universal neonatal screening has a lower running cost and much lower cost per child detected than HVDT.'

(Davis *et al.*, 1997:iii)

value considered. If the derivation of evidence is not clear, then we must harbour doubts about its validity (Humphris, 1999).

A major attribute of evidence should be that it is reliable. If we can't rely on nursing activities and interventions to produce the desired effect, then their use becomes highly questionable. Ziman (1978:6) identified two important attributes of reliable knowledge: not only should it be public, but it should also be consensable and consensual. Consensability means that the evidence is widely and uniformly understood. It should not be so obscure that the potential user cannot either agree or make well-founded objections. Consensuality means that there is general agreement on the implications of the evidence, in that it consists of well-established facts or principles, which are widely accepted without any serious doubt. In relation to neonatal hearing screening, it may be argued that consensability and consensuality are currently being realized (Hind *et al.*, 2001).

Critics of the EBH movement have often expressed anxiety about its dismissive attitude towards the importance of personal experience (*see*, for example, Clarke, 1999). This is a misunderstanding. The third key element in the definition above is the clear statement that best evidence must be integrated with individual clinical expertise. Such expertise is essential to the delivery of excellent nursing care, but it is not evidence. To conflate clinical expertise with evidence is to devalue the importance of individual experience, by obscuring it under an inappropriate category.

The definition above identifies reliable evidence as that produced by systematic research. The kind of evidence, which, according to this definition, does not come under the aegis of EBN, includes anything that does not provide convincing grounds for belief. This includes, for example, personal opinion and anecdote. Neither of these can be scrutinized by any member of the public for information about how they were derived. However, not all are agreed on this point. There are other forms of evidence that are also used in nursing practice and need to be considered. For example, Le May (1999:2) suggested that there is a rather different, more extensive range of kinds of evidence that inform practice, including:

1. Evidence from research (either our own or others').
2. Evidence based on experiences (professional and general).
3. Evidence based on theory that is not research based.
4. Evidence gathered from clients/patients and/or their carers.
5. Evidence passed on by role models/experts.
6. Evidence based on policy directives.

I would not disagree that all six of these are used by nurses, singly and in combination, both appropriately and otherwise. However, if the definition of evidence presented at the beginning of this chapter is accepted, i.e. evidence provides 'ground for belief . . . to prove or disprove any conclusion', then not all can be considered to be forms of evidence. Some are convincing and others may or may not be. Let us consider each of these.

Evidence from research (either our own or others')

The systematic nature of research should ensure that findings can be used by the wider nursing community with reasonable confidence. All research has shortcomings; so critical appraisal skills are needed in order to decide whether or not the quality of research is sufficient to support the conclusions drawn from it. All nurses should be able to appraise and use research, as Department of Health policy (Department of Health, 1999a, 2000a) identifies as a key objective: 'to help the nursing profession to better use research-informed and research-evaluated evidence to support professional practice' (Department of Health, 2000a:2).

A minority of nurses are, and will be, involved in undertaking research and contributing to the evidence base for practice. Those who wish to be involved in research need to have the appropriate training and support (in the same way that we learn the skills of nursing). The numbers of practising community-based nurses involved in undertaking research will always be small, but the need for opportunities for nurses to develop those skills has been recognized (NHS Executive, 1997; Department of Health, 2000a). Schemes such as the Department of Health-funded career scientist awards for those in primary care are, for example, aimed at developing the community nurse research leaders of the future (Department of Health, 1999b; www.doh.gov.uk/research/rd1/pcdevelopmentprog.htm). Primary-care research and development networks cover much of the UK providing the opportunity for practitioners interested in research to obtain support and advice from like-minded colleagues and to access training and project funding (Hungin and Rubin, 2001). Local schemes also support the development of research skills amongst primary health care practitioners (Bryar and Bytheway, 1996).

Evidence based on experiences (professional and general)

Use of this type of evidence involves reflection on one's own and others' experiences, including published patient case-studies. Reflection on experience has become a more explicit element in nursing practice in recent years (see Chapter 2). There is little doubt that the most excellent nurses are almost always those with the greatest experience. Years of experience can tune nurses in to the most subtle cues from patients, which allow rapid and expert care to be delivered (MacLeod, 1994). These may be missed by less-experienced nurses. Experienced nurses can often predict problems and needs, which other nurses could not, allowing for early intervention.

However, experience is not always a guarantee of excellent practice. Even experienced nurses in many arenas hold personal opinions, which have no factual basis. For example, many have firm beliefs about the amount of pain certain conditions 'should' cause. A district nurse's experience may suggest that leg ulcers, for example, cause discomfort rather than overt pain. There is evidence to suggest that, for many, this condition is in fact extremely painful, and that some sufferers have even considered suicide as a result (Briggs, unpublished data, 1999). Obviously, poorly grounded personal opinions of this kind can lead to inappropriate care and much unnecessary suffering. While experience is undoubtedly of great value, it is not always reliable.

Evidence based on theory that is not research based

Le May (1999:3) suggested that this: 'involves searching the literature (published and unpublished), learning from others (for instance in formal education) and facilitating discussion'. All of us have learned much from the ideas of others and through discussion and reflection. It would be hoped that much learned through formal education would be research-based nowadays, and that theory would be used to stimulate thinking rather than provide evidence. Even though much useful information can be gained this way, theory is just theory, and needs to be tested and validated in the real world before being widely accepted. For example, the *National Service Framework for Older People* (Department of Health, 2001a) identifies the prevention of falls as a key area for action. We may have a theory that if we can provide older people with hip protection, this will be the best way to reduce their incidence of hip fracture. Searching the literature will identify that research has been undertaken on this subject and Box 3.2 provides some information from the Cochrane Review on the use of hip protectors (Parker *et al.*, 2001).

This evidence shows that support for our theory is mixed. In particular, the review makes clear that it is difficult to generalize results from studies undertaken in nursing homes, residential homes or schemes supporting people at home to the general population of older people in the community, with whom nurses and health visitors are in contact. That discomfort and practicality reduced the acceptability of hip protectors illustrates the importance of patient preference in the success or otherwise of an intervention.

The national service framework (NSF) and other guidance for primary-care teams and local health groups (National Osteoporosis Society, 1999) indicate that the strategy, for the general population of older people, should address the prevention of falling and the reduction of impact through prevention of osteoporosis, rather than the introduction of a mechanical device to reduce the impact of the fall. Reference to such literature may enable us to be more effective in practice by focusing on theories well supported by evidence.

The research base for nursing is expanding, but there is still much practice that may or may not have been subjected to empirical testing. While in many cases this

---

Box 3.2 Evidence of the effectiveness of hip protectors in preventing hip fractures in older people

Background: Hip fracture in the elderly is usually the result of a simple fall. Hip protectors have been advocated as a means to reduce the risk of sustaining a fracture in a fall on the hip.

Selection criteria: All randomised or quasi-randomised controlled trials comparing the use of hip protectors with a control group.

Reviewer's conclusions: Hip protectors appear to reduce the risk of hip fracture within a selected population at high risk of sustaining a hip fracture. The generalisation of the results is unknown beyond a high-risk population. Cost effectiveness is unclear. Results from ongoing trials may clarify this situation. Acceptability by users of the protectors remains a problem, due to discomfort and practicality.

(Parker *et al.*, 2001:1)

may be of little consequence for treatments that are at best ineffective but harmless, but at worst they may be expensive and harmful.

Evidence gathered from clients/patients and/or their carers

This type of evidence, as described by Le May (1999), consists of feedback from carers and clients/patients receiving nursing care, through audit, satisfaction surveys or research. While these types of information are a crucial aspect of evidence-based nursing, I would argue that this is information integrated through clinical expertise and patients' preferences, rather than evidence (as it has been defined here). Information elicited by nurses from patients and carers is generally obtained in three ways: first from other documentation, such as medical records; second, through careful questioning and the noting of other subtle cues (clinical expertise) and third, through audit (feedback from patients and/or carers).

Audit may be used to check that patients/carers have received and are satisfied with the provision and timeliness of their care. Usually audit is used to compare consumers' views with predetermined standards, so that any deficits in care provision can be rectified.

This type of evidence is also found in the writings of people with particular conditions, which can provide insight not available in any other ways. Diamond (1998) has provided a very telling account of his experience of having cancer from the time of diagnosis, which included having a CT scan:

> The great thing about the CT scan is that it looks just like prime-time viewers think the medicine of the future ought to look like: white, clean, non-invasive. Press a button and five minutes later you have an instant picture of just what's wrong with the patient. Just like *Star Trek*.
>
> For five minutes read half an hour, lying stock-still with your head stuck in the machine's cavity, for non-invasive read a syringe full of gunk, which heats up the bloodstream and leaves a nasty taste in the mouth. For instant read when they've got somebody to interpret the results.
>
> And for reassuring – which all of this was meant to be – imagine the hypochondriac claustrophobe lying with his head enclosed in white enamelled metal, seriously considering cancer for the first time.
>
> (from *C: Because Cowards get Cancer too* by John Diamond, published by Vermilion. Reprinted by permission of The Random House Group Ltd.)

Issues identified by patients/clients and carers in these ways can then be investigated further by research. Research can identify best practice, and this evidence should be used to complement the skilled and important knowledge of their situation provided by patients and carers. For example, Brown et al. (2001) have provided a review of the research concerning the different types of knowledge that patients and carers, as opposed to professionals, bring to the care of an older person, which supports the model of 'carers as experts'. They argue that acknowledgement of this role, and its development over time, by health professionals is supported by varying partner relationships between carers and professionals, which enhance the care of the older person (Brown et al., 2001). The knowledge that the individual with a chronic disease has about their condition is the basis for the Expert Patient initiative (Wilson, 2000; Department of Health, 2001b). This initiative is concerned with providing adequate support to individuals to enhance their self-management and is a service development of particular relevance to district nurses.

Information from clients/patients and carers is collected through research using a whole range of research designs, from the randomized controlled trial to ethnographic and action research. The role of consumers in health care research is recognized as being of increasing importance, not only as sources of data but also as generators of research questions, designers of research, managers of research studies and contributors to evaluation processes (Hanley, 2001) (*see* Chapters 5 and 12). This may help to ensure that research undertaken is more relevant to the actual clinical needs of clients and consumers and, thus, that the services developed based on this research are more appropriate to their needs.

Evidence passed on by role models/experts

Such evidence may be available in the workplace and in the research literature. In the workplace a senior member of staff, such as a district nursing team leader, may act as a role model to more junior nurses, passing on evidence or anecdotes from their experience. Le May (1999) suggests that research in the form of Delphi surveys, which involve a number of experts in coming to agreement on the definition or meaning of the issue being investigated, provides another example of this type of evidence. Delphi surveys are undertaken when there is a lack of consensus on an issue. For example, Beech (2001) describes a number of Delphi studies, including one by Walker *et al.* (2000) which was concerned with gaining an understanding of the role required of mental health nurses in primary care from the perspectives of community psychiatric nurses (CPN), GPs, social workers, service managers and purchasers. Three rounds were undertaken with the panel and the findings were then tested with a sample of users. The conclusion was that there was a need for mental health nurse consultants in the community to supplement the role of the CPN by acting as a therapist, consultant/educator advisor, undertaking assessments and acting in a liaison role between primary care and other services.

Role models and experts no doubt have much to offer, but their opinions do not necessarily constitute reliable evidence. For example, if you think of three of your experienced colleagues and you asked them to discuss the future of public health nursing, you might well get three completely different views. They may or may not draw on research evidence to support those views – but convincing research evidence would be a persuasive addition to the argument. It is not unknown for the charisma of role models to convince, rather than the content of their argument. However, if a *group* of experts comes to a consensus about a question, this would be far more convincing, and of considerable value where no systematically obtained evidence is available. Indeed, as shown later in Table 3.2, this source of evidence appears in the hierarchy of evidence as the weakest type, only resorted to when other stronger types of evidence are unavailable.

Such a group of experts has reviewed the question as to whether health visitors should provide a universal service, to all families, or should be providing a targeted

---

Box 3.3 Universal versus targeted health visiting

Summary points:

- The bulk of problems in society arise in the many people who are not at especially high risk, rather than the few who are at high risk. Consequently, the provision of targeted or selective services will leave untouched a vast burden of health and social problems.
- Within a universally provided service, some clients will require a greater intensity of input in order to derive the maximum benefit from the service.
- Where interventions are most effective among those at greatest risk, the provision of universal services may reduce inequalities in health.
- No screening instrument can be sufficiently precise or accurate to identify those at greatest risk. The professional judgements of health visitors are crucial to an assessment of the need for services.

(Elkan *et al.*, 2000:249)

---

service to families identified as having greater needs. The research evidence in the UK supporting universal or targeted visiting to families is not available. An expert group undertook a review of the available information on this issue and, on the basis of this and their own experience, reached the conclusion that universal was more effective that targeted health visiting, as shown in Box 3.3.

Such consensus amongst experts provides a basis for practice and policy until systematic research on this aspect of health visiting in the UK is available.

Anecdotes, similarly to professional opinion, provide an unreliable source of evidence. For example, a district nurse tells a student about a patient she had visited 2 years earlier who was miraculously cured of long-term headaches once the nurse had persuaded her to drink more fresh orange juice. There is no reason to assume that there is a causal link between the two. More water might have had the same effect, or the patient might have started taking paracetamol that day, unbeknown to the nurse. Or the headaches might have stopped because her family circumstances improved, or she won the lottery! This kind of anecdote should not be used as a basis for future action, although anecdotes such as this may be a rich source for research questions.

Evidence based on policy directives

Policy directives may or may not be based on the type of evidence included in the definition given at the beginning of this chapter. Until recently, NHS policy has rarely been based on research. For example, over the years policy has regularly changed concerning where health care should be delivered – changing from centralized, hospital-based care to dispersed, community-based care and back again. Little research evidence has been produced to support either approach. Nurses and other practitioners working in community and primary care have experienced a number of policy changes for which there was little or no evidence. The introduction of GP fund holding, which led to massive changes in the work of many health care practitioners, is frequently cited as a policy initiative unsupported by research evidence (Meads and Meads, 2001).

By contrast, the introduction recently of national service frameworks provides an example of policy guidance that is soundly rooted in research evidence. As shown in Box 3.4 the practice and policy standards described are supported by the relevant evidence, which may be accessed by patients and professionals.

Box 3.4 Extract from the coronary heart disease NSF

Heart failure

Standard eleven: Doctors should arrange for people with suspected heart failure to be offered appropriate investigations (e.g. electrocardiography, echocardiography) that will confirm or refute the diagnosis. For those in whom heart failure is confirmed, its cause should be identified – the treatments most likely to both relieve symptoms and reduce their risk of death should be offered.

Rationale – prognosis

6. Heart failure often has a poor prognosis, with survival rates worse than those for breast and prostate cancer (Sanderson, 1994). Despite grading heart failure by severity of symptoms, it is difficult to specify a prognosis for people with heart failure as they have a high risk of sudden death. There are thought to be about 6000 deaths a year due to heart failure associated with CHD (Cowie et al., 1997). Annual mortality for those with heart failure ranges from 10 per cent to over 50 per cent depending on severity (CONSENSUS trial study group, 1987).

7. There is evidence that people with heart failure have a worse quality of life than people with most other common medical conditions. Psychosocial function is impaired with over a third experiencing severe and prolonged depressive illness. (Lynn et al., 1997; Sharpe and Doughty, 1998).

Evidence

Cowie MR, Mosterd, Wood D et al. (1997) The epidemiology of heart failure. *European Heart Journal* 18: 208–25.

Lynn J, Harrell F, Cohn F et al. (1997) Prognoses of seriously ill hospitalised patients on the days before death: implications for patient care and public policy. *New Horizons* 5: 56–61.

Sanderson S 1994 ACE Inhibitors in the treatment of chronic heart failure: effective and cost effective. *Bandolier* 1(8): 8–10.

Sharpe N and Doughty R 1998 Epidemiology of heart failure and ventricular dysfunction. *Lancet* 352(1): 3–7.

The CONSENSUS trial study group 1987 Effects of enalapril on mortality in severe congestive heart failure: results of the co-operative north Scandinavian enalapril study. (CONSENSUS). *New England Journal of Medicine* 316: 1429–35.

(Department of Health, 2000b:2–3)

Secondary reporting of research evidence

This last item was not in Le May's list, but is worth a mention. Press cuttings, from the national press or nursing weeklies, should always be read with a pinch of salt. The press want to grab their readers' attention, so use modes of reporting that may be highly misleading. Current examples of such stories may be found in the National electronic Library for Health (NeLH). As the example in Box 3.5 shows, the Library provides information on the use of the story in the press and other media and provides information on the research or other sources for the story.

In this example the press reports suggested that the trial was about the treatment of urinary tract infections whereas the trial was actually about the *prevention of recurrent* urinary tract infections. The headline in a professional journal on the other hand gave the impression that the juice would prevent infections occurring: 'Cranberry juice reduces urinary tract infections although this impression was corrected in the first sentence of the item (Clinical News, 2001). However, in addition, the NeLH review of the original research article (*see* Box 3.5) suggests that there were problems in the conduct of the study including problems in recruiting enough subjects and ensuring that they complied with taking the drink, which weaken the results. As illustrated here secondary reporting virtually always misses out such information, which is needed for an accurate appraisal of the evidence and omission of which may misrepresent the conclusions of the researchers.

Box 3.5 The efficacy of cranberry juice

Two newspapers (1, 2) report on 29 June 2001 that cranberry juice may help to clear urinary tract infections in women. Both incorrectly state that the study confirms the effectiveness of cranberry juice as a 'cure' for urinary tract infections. The study actually looks at the 'prevention' of urinary tract infections.

Overall, the trial suggests that cranberry juice may be beneficial in the prevention of recurrent urinary tract infections in women. However, the findings should be treated with caution. The trial fails to determine the long-term effectiveness of drinking cranberry juice, given that women may be susceptible to recurrent infections over a very long period of time.

References

1. Cranberry juice clears infection. *The Guardian* 29 June 2001: 7.
2. Efficacy of cranberry juice. *The Financial Times* 29 June 2001: 4.
3. Kontiokari T, Sundqvist K, Nuutinen M, Pokka T, Koskela M, Uhari M 2001 Randomised trial of cranberry–lingonberry juice and *Lactobacillus* GG drink for the prevention of urinary tract infections in women. *BMJ* 322: 1571–5.

(http://www.nelh.nhs.uk/hth/cranberry.asp; accessed 4 July 2001)

Evidence: A summary

In summary, these seven types of 'evidence' are different from the type of evidence produced by external systematic research. All have a place in clinical practice and are sources of information routinely used by nurses. The remainder of this chapter is concerned with understanding how use may be made in practice of the most reliable evidence that is available, as defined at the beginning of this chapter.

There is one final and important reason for accepting that research is the main component of what we should consider to be reliable evidence: this view concurs with the use of the word by other professionals with whom nurses work closely. Effective change strategies are facilitated by a shared language, which has the same meaning for nurses, GPs and other health care practitioners with whom they work (*see* Chapter 4). If a community nursing team, or the wider primary health care team, is going to effectively introduce evidence-based changes into the care of patients, it is important that they are all speaking the same language.

EVIDENCE-BASED NURSING: WHAT IT IS

The practice of evidence-based nursing depends not only on the availability and quality of evidence and the clinical expertise of the nurse, but also individual patient preferences within the resources available (Fig. 3.1). Figure 3.1 illustrates the place of evidence in underpinning the nurse–patient interaction. Figure 3.2 provides an example of the interrelationship of the four elements in relation to supporting an individual to give up smoking. The research evidence supporting smoking cessation strategies is provided in Box 3.6.

It is clear from Fig. 3.2 that where there is a lack of congruence, for example in the practitioners' skills, the person's readiness to change or in the adequacy of the evidence, then the resultant change in the behaviour of the individual is likely to be affected.

The nurse's expertise and the patient's requirements may make it inappropriate to use the best evidence in every case. For example, while evidence shows that heavy smoking is detrimental to health, an alcoholic who is in the process of giving up drinking may find it impossible to give up smoking at the same time. Similarly, while there is evidence of the benefit of a low-fat diet for those with hypertension, changes in diet might not be the main priority for the carer of a spouse with dementia who is found by the practice nurse to be hypertensive. In such cases it is unlikely that a nurse would push the 'best evidence' line, since it would be likely to result in greater problems for the client, at least in the short term.

The whole enterprise of evidence-based nursing takes place according to the resources available. This includes all three of the factors shown within Fig. 3.1. The best possible care takes place in the area where the three circles overlap. An interesting exercise would be to draw similar diagrams for the care of different people or communities with whom you are involved. The ideal would be to achieve completely coterminous circles.

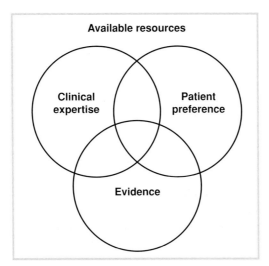

Fig. 3.1 *Essential elements of evidence-based nursing.*

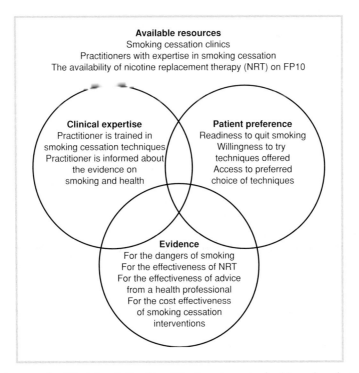

Fig. 3.2 *An example of the interrelationship of the four elements of evidence-based nursing: smoking cessation.*

Box 3.6 Evidence supporting smoking cessation strategies and evidence-based nursing

Agency for Health Care Policy and Research 1996 *Smoking cessation. Clinical practice guideline.* Agency for Health Care Policy and Research, Rockville, USA.

Buck D, Godfrey C, Parrott S and Raw R 1997 *Cost effectiveness of smoking cessation interventions.* Health Education Authority, London.

Cromwell J, Bartosch WJ, Fiore MC *et al.* 1997 Cost-effectiveness of the clinical practice recommendations in the AHCPR guideline for smoking cessation. *JAMA* 278: 1759–66.

Doll R, Peto R, Wheatley K *et al.* 1994 Mortality in relation to smoking: 40 years' observations on male British doctors. *BMJ* 309: 901–11.

Law M, Ling Tang J 1995 An analysis of the effectiveness of interventions intended to help people stop smoking. *Archives of Internal Medicine* 155: 1933–1941.

Ling Tang J, Law M, Wald N 1994 How effective is nicotine replacement therapy in helping people to stop smoking? *BMJ* 308: 21–6.

Peto R, Lopez AD, Boreham J *et al.* 1992 Mortality from tobacco in developed countries: indirect estimation from national vital statistics. *Lancet* 339: 1268–70.

Silagy C, Ketteridge S 1998 Physician advice for smoking cessation. In: Lancaster T, Silagy C, Fullerton D (Eds) *Tobacco Addiction Module of the Cochrane Database of Systematic Reviews.* Available in The Cochrane Library (database on disk and CD-ROM). The Cochrane Collaboration; Issue 1. Update Software, Oxford.

Silagy C, Mant D, Fowler G, Lancaster T 1998 Nicotine replacement therapy for smoking cessation. In: Lancaster T, Silagy C, Fullerton D (Eds) *Tobacco Addiction Module of the Cochrane Database of Systematic Reviews.* Available in The Cochrane Library (database on disk and CD-ROM). The Cochrane Collaboration; Issue 1. Update Software, Oxford.

Warner KE 1997 Cost effectiveness of smoking-cessation therapies: interpretation of the evidence and implications for coverage. *Pharmacoeconomics* 11: 538–49.

Evidence

Questions from and about practice and care of the client/patient constitute the starting point for the identification of evidence to provide answers to the questions (Flemming, 1998). Starting out with a clear, structured answerable question is key to the whole process. The carefully constructed questions can then be used to guide literature searching, so that relevant, external evidence can be identified. Library resources are needed in order to obtain research and other published evidence. Access to databases such as Best Evidence, the Cochrane Library (including databases of systematic reviews and controlled trials), Cinahl, Medline and PsycINFO are useful, as well as to up-to-date journals. Time is a crucial resource which is needed to access this kind of information.

The NHS Centre for Reviews and Dissemination at the University of York produces *Effective Health Care* bulletins, which summarize all the available evidence on a particular topic – these are particularly useful and time saving. Journals such as *Evidence-Based Nursing* contain brief summaries of recently published research studies together with critical commentaries on those studies, which can also save busy nurses considerable time (*see* Chapter 12).

Clinical expertise

The presence of experienced nurses, and co-operative colleagues both within and outside nursing, is a requirement for best possible care. Their direct clinical expertise includes a wide range of disparate skills, which might loosely be grouped around assessment, intervention and evaluation. Wider skills may also be needed to implement research findings (*see* Chapter 4). Organization, management and communication skills are essential to the success of this enterprise. These abilities might improve the chances of persuading the board of a Primary Care Trust to spend money on new services such as screening, when research is published which suggests that it is effective. Nurses also need the ability to communicate effectively with patients and their carers about the risks and benefits of different options for care. The traditional view of what constitutes clinical expertise might be extended to include the ability to seek evidence efficiently, and to possess critical appraisal skills.

Patient preferences

The preferences of patients in terms of care will depend on a range of resources. These might include specific types of dressing or back support, or aspects of diet such as the cost of different foods versus personal taste and possible benefits. Someone at risk of heart disease might be unable to take much exercise, for example, in which case other lifestyle changes could be a focus instead.

Available resources

The resources needed to support evidence-based practice are of several different kinds. They include the availability of and access to library resources; finances to support new equipment; an adequate number of nurses with an adequate skill mix; time for gathering and appraising evidence; time for implementation activities; and co-operation from peers, managers and other professionals. There is evidence that access to these resources proves difficult for many nurses and health visitors working in community and primary care.

A study was undertaken in three community trusts and one health authority area to identify the barriers that prevent nurses using research evidence in practice (Griffiths *et al.*, 2001). Data were collected from all nurses and health visitors working in the community and from practice nurses in primary care. A response rate of 51.5 per cent was achieved. As shown in Table 3.1, the respondents from the four settings all identified time as the greatest barrier to the use of research. Practice nurses found the amount of research overwhelming and also had greater difficulties with lack of co-operation by doctors in charge than did the respondents in the community trusts. Those in trusts found inadequacies in the facilities and difficulties with understanding statistical analysis greater barriers, along with a feeling in one trust of a personal lack of authority to change practice.

In summary, it is apparent that evidence-based nursing in the community requires both individual nurses and their patients to be aware of best evidence and

Table 3.1 *Percentage of sample who rated barriers as moderate to great according to setting (values in bold are the top three barriers for each sub-sample)*

Item	All	Trust 1	Trust 2	Trust 3	Practice nurses
1. Research reports are not readily available	47.6	44.3	44.3	53.3	40.3
2. Implications for practice are not made clear	52.0	50.1	50.3	55.0	48.1
3. Statistical analysis is not understandable	**66.2**	60.9	**67.0**	**69.4**	63.6
4. The research is not relevant to the nurse's practice	35.7	35	34.3	36.3	41.6
5. The nurse is unaware of the research	58.1	51.9	55.7	63.9	58.4
6. The facilities are inadequate for implementation	**66.5**	**65.9**	**65.4**	**67.7**	66.2
7. The nurse does not have time to read research	63.1	61.8	62.2	65.9	54.5
8. The research has not been replicated	45.6	47	43.2	46.9	42.7
9. The nurse feels the benefits of changing practice will be minimal	32.4	34.1	33.0	30.4	35.1
10. The nurse is uncertain whether to believe the results of the research	41.7	44.3	40.5	41.2	39.0
11. The research has methodological inadequacies	40.6	45.2	41.4	35.7	48.1
12. The relevant literature is not compiled in one place	62.6	56.5	62.7	66.7	62.3
13. The nurse does not feel she/he has enough authority to change patient care procedures	58.5	**62.7**	56.5	58.4	50.6
14. The nurse feels results are not generalizable to own setting	56.3	58.6	56.3	54	61
15. The nurse is isolated from knowledgeable colleagues with whom to discuss the research	52.0	46.9	44.3	60.9	53.2
16. The nurse sees little benefit for self	28.1	27.7	27.8	28.8	27.3
17. Research reports/articles are not published fast enough	33.5	36.7	34.6	29.2	41.6
18. Doctors will not co-operate with implementation	54.0	58.0	56.5	47.1	**70.1**
19. Administration will not allow implementation	42.3	45.5	46.8	35.1	53.2
20. The nurse does not see the value of research for practice	18.9	18.1	19.2	20.3	11.7
21. There is not a documented need to change practice	22.7	24.5	19.5	23.7	24.7
22. The conclusions drawn from the research are not justified	23.4	28.6	23.5	19.9	23.4
23. The literature reports conflicting results	47.8	50.4	51.6	42.6	51.9
24. The research is not reported clearly and readably	58.5	59.5	61.9	55.6	57.1
25. Other staff are not supportive of implementation	54.4	52.4	50.8	58	57.1
26. The nurse is unwilling to change/try new ideas	29.9	29.2	29.7	32.7	15.6
27. The amount of research information is overwhelming	59.2	57.7	61.6	56.5	**71.4**
28. The nurse does not feel capable of evaluating the quality of the research	56.2	52.8	56.8	58.8	51.9
29. There is insufficient time on the job to implement new ideas	**71.9**	**67.3**	**71.9**	**74.6**	**75.3**

an organizational context, including supportive colleagues and access to resources, which is open to change.

BEST EVIDENCE?

The preceding section has argued that the nature of the evidence needed in evidence-based nursing is, for the most part, of the kinds cited by Muir Gray (1997) and others, as shown in Table 3.2.

This hierarchy indicates, in a very approximate way, how convincing is each of these levels of evidence. It works well for medicine, which has a long history and an enormous body of research, and in particular randomized controlled trials, to support it. The kinds of intervention which medicine uses tend to be of a discrete, easily defined nature, such as drugs and particular types of surgery. These are far easier to control and evaluate than many nursing interventions, and are, therefore, far more amenable to assessment using controlled trials.

The picture is rather different for nursing (and in other disciplines in primary health care), however. As an academic discipline, it is less than half a century old. Consequently, we do not have large numbers of trials to extract evidence from; indeed much of the available research is exploratory. This is entirely to be expected at this stage of our development – exploratory work is a necessary precursor to more evaluative work, and, of course, some of it stands in its own right. And, as was implied earlier, many nursing interventions could not be controlled sufficiently in order to subject them to evaluation using a randomized controlled trial.

Examination of the hierarchy shows that qualitative research is not included. Qualitiative research approaches are important but they are not part of the 'effectiveness' paradigm. Qualitative research does not seek causal inferences. Rather, it develops theory upon which various aspects of nursing may draw.

Qualitative findings tend (although not exclusively) to be used in one of three ways. First, they may stand alone in generating a testable theory, which may then be subjected to further research. Second, when qualitative data are elicited alongside

Table 3.2   *Strength of different types of evidence*

Type	Strength of evidence
I	Strong evidence from at least one systematic review of multiple well-designed randomized controlled trials
II	Strong evidence from at least one properly designed randomized controlled trial of appropriate size
III	Evidence from well-designed trials without randomization, single group pre-post, cohort, time series or matched case-control studies
IV	Evidence from well-designed non-experimental studies from more than one centre or research group
V	Opinions of respected authorities, based on clinical evidence, descriptive studies or reports of expert committees

Source: NHS Centre for Reviews and Dissemination, 1996.

quantitative data, they complement and supplement it, helping to explain and add depth to what may otherwise be oversimplistic findings. Third, they may inform nurses' thinking, by challenging entrenched norms and individual perspectives. The lack of generalizability (credibility, transferability or whatever term is preferred to label this basic concept) means that qualitative findings cannot be used to make widespread changes to nursing care in settings beyond those of the study from which they are derived. Instead, they may add to how nurses think about those they care for, broadening and deepening their understanding or perhaps their sensitivity to issues of which they might previously have been unaware.

There has, as just alluded to, been a long-standing (and rather tedious) debate in nursing about whether qualitative or quantitative research provides the 'best' evidence for nursing practice. Hunt (1997) rightly identified this as time wasted, and as a barrier to 'research-mindedness' in nursing. Indeed, it is a vacuous debate, since the approach taken to research depends on the question being asked – and there are huge numbers of questions of all kinds that nursing needs to ask about its own practice. All methods have something valuable to offer, provided they are undertaken scientifically.

Another tedious debate is concerned with the debunking of positivism, which for some obscure reason is often assumed to be synonymous with science. Both science and positivism have been regarded with great suspicion in the nursing literature. They are not synonymous. Positivism was a movement that assumed (amongst other things) that absolute truths could be found, a position with clear limitations, and the movement faded in the 1960s. The repeated pillorying of positivism is understandable, but a waste of time. It is setting up a straw man, which can easily be knocked down. Science, on the other hand, is fundamental to our thinking about evidence-based nursing practice. The most compelling definition I have come across was proposed by the physicist John Ziman (1998:28): '[Science is] A peculiar type of social institution, devoted to the production of public, communally acceptable knowledge about the natural and social worlds through a delicately balanced tension between originality and criticism'.

This approach to generating knowledge can equally be subsumed within any research method, qualitative, quantitative or in between – provided that it is undertaken systematically and with rigour, and is reported transparently.

Best evidence available?

Systematic reviews currently provide the best, most comprehensive evidence on specific topics. The NHS Centre for Reviews and Dissemination at the University of York provides a focus for much of this work, and produces free publications resulting from these reviews. *Effective Health Care* bulletins are produced bi-monthly. Each of these is based on a systematic review of a particular topic, which synthesizes all relevant research on the clinical effectiveness, cost effectiveness and acceptability of health care interventions.

There is a limited number of reviews available, but many of those published to date are relevant to nurses working in the community (Box 3.7).

Minimal critical appraisal skills are needed in order to use the results of system-

---

Box 3.7 Relevant topics covered by *Effective Health Care* bulletins

- The treatment of depression in primary care (Vol. 1, No. 5).
- Implementing clinical practice guidelines (Vol. 1, No. 8).
- Preventing falls and subsequent injury in older people (Vol. 2, No. 4).
- Preventing unintentional injuries in children and young adolescents (Vol. 2, No. 5).
- Preventing and reducing the adverse effects of unintended teenage pregnancies (Vol. 3, No. 1).
- The prevention and treatment of obesity (Vol. 3, No. 2).
- Mental health promotion in high-risk groups (Vol. 3, No. 3).
- Compression therapy for venous leg ulcers (Vol. 3, No. 4).
- Cholesterol and coronary heart disease: screening and treatment (Vol. 4, No. 1).
- Pre-school hearing, speech, language and vision screening (Vol. 4, No. 2).
- Deliberate self-harm (Vol. 4, No. 6).
- Getting evidence into practice (Vol. 5, No. 1).
- Preventing the uptake of smoking in young people (Vol. 5, No. 5).
- Promoting the initiation of breastfeeding (Vol. 6, No. 2).
- Acute and chronic low back pain (Vol. 6, No. 5).
- Counselling in primary care (Vol. 6, No. 7).

---

atic reviews, since they are undertaken by research teams with advice from expert consultants and subject to extensive and rigorous peer review. Indeed, the aim of the *Effective Health Care* bulletins is to summarize the 'state of the art' on specific topics in order to inform health care professionals in a way that minimizes the time and effort spent on obtaining the information. Even so, it is always wise to maintain a healthily sceptical attitude towards all such publications. Indeed, there are guidelines available for appraising systematic reviews (*see*, for example, Muir Gray 1997:74–7 and the workbook on evidence-based practice by Greenhalgh and Donald, 2000).

One of the most important questions to ask of such reviews is: is it answering the question I am interested in? For example, an *Effective Heath Care* bulletin has been produced on breastfeeding (NHS Centre for Reviews and Dissemination, 2000). For many midwives and health visitors the main question they are interested in concerning breastfeeding is: What interventions help women to continue breastfeeding after the first few days or weeks? The *Effective Health Care* bulletin, however, does not look at this question but is concerned with the initiation of breastfeeding and: ' . . . reviews the evidence for the effectiveness of interventions to increase the *initiation* of breastfeeding' (NHS Centre for Reviews and Dissemination, 2000:1) (italics added). While this is an important question, this review cannot help answer questions about continuation of breastfeeding and demonstrates the need to look carefully at the focus of a systematic review.

Of course, not all topics of interest to community-based nurses, midwives and health visitors have been subjected to systematic review. Many topics will require literature searching and critical appraisal skills. These skills are key to the identification of valid and clinically usable evidence. Indeed, much of the evidence-based health care movement nationwide has focused on critical appraisal without always considering the wider issues involved in changing practice.

The intricacies of how research reports should be read critically and appraised will not be considered here. However, an excellent book that presents the appraisal of different kinds of research very accessibly is: *How to read a paper: the basics of evidence based medicine*, by Tricia Greenhalgh (2001). Don't be put off by the word 'medicine' appearing in the title, since it is equally suitable for most members of the health care professions. The workbook based on the first edition of this book enables individuals and groups to apply the process of critical appraisal (Greenhalgh and Donald, 2000). The management of change is discussed elsewhere in this book (*see* Chapter 4).

Community issues

It's all very well presenting an idealized version of evidence-based nursing, as designed for hospital-based nurses with access to many resources. In a primary care setting there are some unique problems (Muir Gray, 1997:167):

1. A wider range of health problems is seen.
2. Primary-care professionals are scattered geographically.
3. Many important decisions have to be made in a patient's home.
4. Access to a library is difficult and the support of a librarian is rarely available.

Although numerous different health problems are dealt with, those that occur frequently are smaller in number. Efforts to obtain evidence may, therefore, be focused on a limited range of fairly specific topics. For example, the sorts of problems concerning under 1-year-olds that health visitors may come across on a regular basis include difficulties with breastfeeding and excessive infant crying. District nurses manage leg ulcers on a regular basis and may frequently be asked for advice about symptom control in terminal care.

The geographical dispersion of primary care professionals is problematic, and is one issue that is likely to benefit from the pooling of multidisciplinary needs and resources. It may be that all Primary Care Trusts will provide educational resource centres in time, providing information points, where key databases, NHS Centre for Reviews and Dissemination reports, guidelines, other material and help in finding evidence will be available.

Making snap decisions in patients' homes may be problematic on occasion. Not only is there the problem of not having key information directly to hand, but there may be pressure from patients and carers to give care considered to be inappropriate by the nurse, or which is beyond the resources available. The boom in information technology, and the increasing access to information via the Internet means that many health care consumers are very well informed. Furthermore, the recent shift in emphasis of the health service to value consumer satisfaction means that health service users have increasingly high expectations of care.

The fourth of these problems is widespread. Difficulty in accessing a library means that computing facilities become essential to those with a community base. Access to databases via the World Wide Web is easily the most convenient and efficient method of identifying evidence. Taking time out to use libraries is probably not feasible for most nurses working in primary care. The Department of Health strategy on the use of IT in the NHS, *Information for Health* (NHS Executive, 1998) has the potential to provide nurses in the community with access to these sources of information, but provision of hardware and training in its use has, to date, not yet given those in the community the benefits that they could utilize in practice development. These and other difficulties contribute to the relatively underdeveloped research culture in community settings.

The 1997 *R&D in Primary Care* report (NHS Executive, 1997) took a more strategic view of the low levels of research and development. The review group set major objectives, including raising the amount of high-quality R&D of importance to NHS primary care; increasing the recruitment, development and retention of R&D leaders in primary care; increasing the number of clinicians with R&D expertise, increasing the involvement of non-clinical disciplines and last (but by no means least) achieving an evidence-based culture in primary care.

Two years later, these objectives were reviewed in the *NHS R&D Strategic Review. Primary Care* (Department of Health, 1999b) and the wider problems of developing research in primary care were also presented. This report contains the recommendations of a multidisciplinary working group, following an assessment of the needs of the service and an identification of evidence gaps in primary care. The gaps identified included:

- A basic science gap – not enough relevant clinical and social research evidence is available.
- An effectiveness gap – effectiveness and cost-effectiveness of care has not been widely assessed.
- An applicability gap – not enough is known about how to apply evidence from clinical trials to specific situations.
- An implementation gap – good evidence about effective care exists, but implementation is poor and patchy.

Several professions, specific and clinical sub-groups contributed to this report, of which one was nursing. This group recommended that four research programmes, each addressing one or more of these gaps, should be taken forward (Department of Health, 1999b:12):

- Evaluating and measuring the effectiveness of primary-care nursing interventions in health maintenance processes of individuals, communities and populations (effectiveness gap).
- Identifying the value-added contribution of nursing to reducing inequalities in health care (effectiveness gap).
- Evaluating different models of assessment and decision-making used in primary care in targeting health inequalities (basic science gap, effectiveness gap and implementation gap).
- Exploration and explanation of the relationship between team-based information sharing and decision making with referral pathways and clinical, professional and organizational outcomes (basic science gap, effectiveness gap and applicability gap).

Furthermore, five multidisciplinary research programmes were proposed, focusing on men's health, mother and infant health, NHS priorities, rehabilitation and therapies, and women's health. There is, not to put too fine a point on it, a vast amount to be done. In the meantime in the community we have to strive to utilize the best available evidence while awaiting systematic research.

CONCLUSION

Evidence-based nursing practice is not a panacea, and at present, skilled researchers and high-quality research are in short supply in the community. Of course, there is some good evidence available. We should, however, be wary of relying on evidence from sources other than high-quality research and expert consensus. But we should also be wary of apparently good evidence from systematic reviews and randomized controlled trials – it may not always be answering the 'right' question.

Alone, evidence-based nursing practice cannot provide the maximum health benefits possible for a population. There are factors outwith the control of the nurse, which have a strong influence on the health of our communities. These include the physical environment, the social environment and lifestyle, and the genetic constitution of individuals. In addition, the degree to which colleagues in other health care professions employ evidence-based practice will impact on health. Last, but not least, the quality of health service management will have a major influence. However, it is only by successfully incorporating evidence-based nursing into everyday practice, with its reliance on high-quality evidence, clinical expertise and patients' preferences, that we can behave professionally, providing the best possible care.

REFERENCES

Beech B 2001 The Delphi approach: recent applications in health care. *Nurse Researcher* 8(4): 38–48.

Briggs A 1972 *Report of the Committee on Nursing.* Cmnd. 5115. HMSO, London.

Brown J, Nolan M and Davies S 2001 Who's the expert? Redefining lay and professional relationships. In: Nolan M, Davies S and Grant G (Eds) *Working with Older People and their Families. Key Issues in Policy and Practice.* Open University Press, Buckingham, pp. 20–32.

Bryar R 1999 Using research in community nursing. In: McIntosh J (Ed.) *Research Issues in Community Nursing.* Macmillan, Basingstoke, pp. 6–28.

Bryar R and Bytheway B 1996 *Changing Primary Health Care. The Teamcare Valleys Experience.* Blackwell Science, Oxford.

Clarke J B 1999 Evidence-based practice: a retrograde step? The importance of pluralism in evidence generation for the practice of health care. *Journal of Clinical Nursing* 8: 89–94.

Clinical News 2001 Cranberry juice reduces urinary tract infections. *Community Practitioner* 74(9): 349.

Davis A, Bamford J, Wilson I, Ramkalawan T, Forshaw M and Wright S 1997 A critical review of the role of neonatal hearing screening in the detection of congenital hearing impairment. *Health Technology Assessment*, Vol. 10, Issue 1.

Department of Health 1999a *Making a Difference: Strengthening the Nursing, Midwifery and Health Visiting Contribution to Health and Healthcare.* Department of Health, London.

Department of Health 1999b *NHS R&D Strategic Review: Primary Care.* (Clarke Report). Department of Health, London.

Department of Health 2000a *Towards a Strategy for Nursing Research and Development*. Proposals for Action. Department of Health, London.

Department of Health 2000b *National Service Frameworks Coronary Heart Disease*. Modern Standards and Service Models. Chapter 6: Heart Failure. Department of Health, London.

Department of Health 2001a *National Service Framework for Older People*. Department of Health, London.

Department of Health 2001b *The Expert Patient: A New Approach to Chronic Disease Management for the 21st Century*. Department of Health, London.

Diamond J 1998 *Because Cowards Get Cancer Too . . . .* Vermillion, London.

Elkan R, Kendrick D, Hewitt M *et al*. 2000 The effectiveness of domiciliary health visiting: a systematic review of international studies and a selective review of the British literature. *Health Technology Assessment*, Vol. 13, Issue 4.

Flemming K 1998 Asking Answerable Questions. *Evidence-Based Nursing* 1(2): 36–7.

Greenhalgh T 2001 *How to Read a Paper: The Basics of Evidence Based Medicine*. BMJ Publishing Group, London.

Greenhalgh T and Donald A 2000 *Evidence Based Health Care Workbook. For Individual and Group Learning*. BMJ Publishing Group, London.

Griffiths J, Bryar R, Closs SJ, Cooke J, Hostick T, Kelly S and Marshall K 2001 Barriers to research implementation identified by community nurses. *British Journal of Community Nursing* 10: 501–10.

Hall DMB (Ed.) 1996 *Health for All Children*, 3rd edition. Oxford University Press, Oxford.

Hanley B 2001 Taking on the Policy Research Programme. *Consumers in NHS Research Support Unit News* Summer: 1.

Hind S, Beresford D, Kimm L, Davis A and Bamford J 2001 National Universal Newborn Hearing Screening. *Community Practitioner*.

Humphris D 1999 Types of evidence. In: Hamer S and Collinson G (Eds) *Achieving Evidence-Based Practice. A Handbook for Practitioners*. Baillière Tindall/RCN Edinburgh, pp. 13–10

Hungin P and Rubin G 2001 Editorial: Are primary care research networks up to the challenge? *Primary Health Care Research and Development* 2(2): 67–8.

Hunt J 1997 Foreword. In: Smith P. (Ed.) *Research Mindedness for Practice. An Interactive Approach for Nursing and Health Care*. Churchill Livingstone, Edinburgh, pp xi–xii.

Le May A 1999 *Evidence-based practice*. Nursing Times Clinical Monograph No. 1. NT Books, London.

MacLeod M 1994 'It's the little things that count': the hidden complexity of everyday clinical nursing practice. *Journal of Clinical Nursing* 3(6): 361–8.

Meads G and Meads T (Eds) 2001 *Trust in Experience. Transferable Learning for Primary Care Trusts*. Radcliffe Medical Press, Abingdon.

Muir Gray JA 1997 *Evidence-based Healthcare. How to Make Health Policy and Management Decisions*. Churchill Livingstone, Edinburgh.

NHS Centre for Reviews and Dissemination 1996 CRD Guidelines for those Carrying Out or Commissioning Reviews. *CRD Report Number 4*, January. University of York, York.

NHS Centre for Reviews and Dissemination 2000 Promoting the initiation of breastfeeding. *Effective Health Care* 6(2).

NHS Executive 1997 *R&D in Primary Care. National Working Group Report*. (Chair Professor D Mant). Department of Health, London.

NHS Executive 1998 *Information for Health. An Information Strategy for the Modern NHS 1998–2005*. NHS Executive, Leeds.

NHS Management Executive 1993 *Nursing in Primary Health Care. New World, New Opportunities.* NHSME, Leeds.

National Osteoporosis Society 1999 *Accidents, Falls, Fractures and Osteoporosis. A Strategy for Primary Care Groups and Local Health Groups.* National Osteoporosis Society, Bath.

Oxford English Dictionary (1994) CD-ROM Version 1.13, 2nd edn. Oxford University Press, Oxford.

Parker MJ, Gillespie LD, Gillespie WJ 2001 *Hip Protectors for Preventing Hip Fractures in the Elderly* (Cochrane Review). Available in The Cochrane Library 3. Update Software, Oxford.

Sackett DL, Rosenberg WMC, Muir Gray JA, Haynes RB and Richardson WS 1996 Evidence-based medicine: What it is and what it isn't. *BMJ* 312:71–2.

Walker L *et al.* 2000 The required role of the psychiatric mental health nurse in primary health care: an augmented delphi study. *Nurse Inquiry* 7: 91–102.

Wilson T 2000 The expert patient: a proactive role for DNs? *British Journal of Community Nursing* 5(5): 212.

Ziman J 1978 *Reliable Knowledge. An Exploration of the Grounds for Belief in Science.* Cambridge University Press, Cambridge.

Ziman J 1998 A limited Excalibur. *The Times Higher Education Supplement* April 24: 25.

4

The process of change: Issues for practice development

Rosamund Bryar and Katrina Bannigan

Purpose of this chapter

- To identify the centrality of change in the process of practice development.
- To examine approaches to change.
- To discuss the application of research findings in practice development.
- To identify factors facilitating the change process.

INTRODUCTION

For all nurses, health visitors and midwives working in primary health and since the early 1990s, change has been an ever-present part of their lives. In a book (entitled tellingly: *Contemporary Primary Care. The Challenges of Change* [Tovey, 2000]) Heywood (2000:26) goes further, in stating that: 'General practice has seen a century of change in service delivery'. As part of the NHS Plan (Department of Health, 2000a), the move to make primary care the central organization in the process of commissioning and providing services has gathered pace, and primary care will soon be responsible for management of 75 per cent of the NHS budget (Department of Health, 2001a). The very purpose of the NHS Plan (Department of Health, 2000a:2) is to bring about change in all aspects of the NHS: 'The NHS Plan sets out the steps we now need to take *to transform* the health service so that it is redesigned around the needs of patients. It means tackling the toughest issues that have been ducked for too long' (our emphasis). And managers and clinicians are charged with bringing about this radical change: 'For every example of good practice there are too many examples where change has yet to take place. Best practice can no longer be an option. Managers and clinicians across the NHS must make change happen' (Department of Health, 2000a:9.2).

In Chapter 2 practice development was defined as follows, based on the NHS Executive definition (NHS Executive, 1998:6): Practice development is work directed towards introducing an innovation or the improvement of a service or process, often based on the findings of research, which also involves evaluation of the innovation or

service development. In Chapter 3 barriers to the application of best evidence in practice were identified, including: the lack of availability of relevant, high-quality research
in primary care; lack of access by community practitioners to the evidence that is available; and lack of skills amongst community practitioners in coming to a judgement
about the quality of the evidence. A fourth factor which has inhibited practice development has been a lack of concern with the process of practice development and change
(Bryar, 1999). As Evans and Haines (2000:xvii) comment, there is a need to: '... address
the imbalance between the growing volume of literature on the theory of evidence-
based practice and the lack of material on implementation based on real world experience'. Greenhalgh (2001) makes the observation that for those intent on introducing
change an additional barrier is the plethora of theories and approaches to change, which
may increase confusion rather than lead to more effective change strategies.

This lack of apparent interest in the process of practice development in primary
health care may reflect an attitude that, as everyone knows about, and is involved in,
change, we all put into practice what we know will achieve effective change. Or it may
reflect a view that change and practice development are too difficult, preventing people from examining the processes involved in detail. Madhok (1999) illustrates these
difficulties from his own experience of the complexities of introducing research findings to affect change in the practice of public health. As shown in Fig. 4.1, his
experience of the change process has led him to identify factors that facilitate change.
These include: the attributes of the person leading the change, i.e. the need for the
facilitator to be flexible, focused and positive; methods of communication, i.e. the
need to make use of formal channels and less formal networks to get the messages of
change across; and the need for sound methods to monitor or evaluate the change
process. As illustrated in Fig. 4.1, the change process involves the need to take an
organizational perspective. The introduction of new knowledge or practices may
have far-reaching impacts on many parts of an organization which can, in their turn,
facilitate or undermine the change process. Most notably perhaps, Madhok identifies
that: 'Change does take a long time' – the same conclusion reached by the authors of
Chapter 10 in their experience of developing a nursing development unit.

Recognition of the need to support the process of implementation of research
findings in the development of practice was highlighted by the Select Committee on
Science and Technology (House of Lords, 1988) and has been reiterated in the
Department of Health (2000b) document: *Towards a Strategy for Nursing Research
and Development*. The final section of the strategy is concerned with this topic and it
is suggested that:

> 24. Greater emphasis is needed on the dissemination and application of research
> findings to practice. There is a need to maximise the impact of research and
> development to ensure that this knowledge is transferred to practice and education.
>
> (Department of Health, 2000b:6)

It is acknowledged that one of the barriers to such implementation is lack of access
to the best available evidence and improved access is advocated '... especially in community and primary care settings...' (Department of Health, 2000b: 6). Another barrier may be lack of awareness of the mechanisms to achieve change, which this chapter

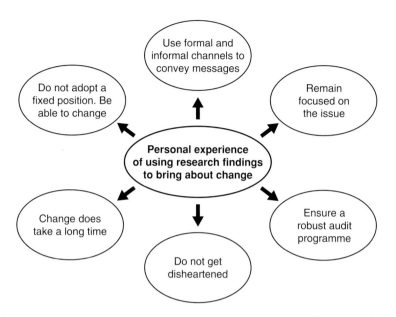

Fig. 4.1 *Learning the lessons 1: A public health practitioner's experience (from Madhok, 1999: 3–7).*

seeks to address. This chapter aims to focus specifically on the process of introduction of: 'an innovation or the improvement of a service or process' (*see* definition above), i.e. to focus on the process of change and approaches to change which may be used within practice development activities.

CHANGE

The definition of change identifies the active nature of this process: 'to alter or make different; to give or receive for another or for an equivalent; to cause to move or pass from one state to another; to exchange or replace' (*Chambers Dictionary*, 1994:285). This definition suggests that the impact of an alteration in a service or clinical practice brought about by change is far reaching, and that this impact may be felt not only by the patients or clients in receipt of the service but by those providing the service. Change, according to Marris (1986) may be of one of three types: sudden and unexpected; revolutionary; or planned. The majority of practice development activities will fall into the category of planned change, although, even with careful preparation, some practice development may be perceived by some as sudden and unexpected. Revolutionary change, implying violence and destruction, is also not a usual approach to practice development.

However, Marris (1986) suggests that consideration of the reaction of individuals to sudden, unexpected or revolutionary change may be helpful when undertaking planned change activities such as practice development. Through research in many different community settings, Marris suggests that reactions to change can be understood in the same way as the reaction of an individual to the bereavement of a close family member or friend. So the community nurse involved in a practice development project may react with anger, threatening and challenging those involved in introducing the change. She might react with despair, feelings of hopelessness and depression and withdraw from communication regarding the development. Alternatively, she may appear to deny that the change is taking place and continue with pre-existing patterns of behaviour.

Like bereavement, Marris (1986:157) considers that change may threaten the picture that individuals have developed of themselves, for example, as competent practitioners:

> Change threatens to invalidate this experience, robbing them of the skills they have learned and confusing their purposes, upsetting the subtle rationalisations and compensations by which they reconciled the different aspects of their situation.

The practitioner faced with evidence that undermines his or her previous practice may react with anger against the new ideas, may question the basis for the changes or provide passive resistance to change through apparently accepting but then taking no action to implement the changes. Many health visitors and midwives probably still have concerns about their own practice prior to the research findings which support the 'Back to Sleep' campaign for babies. Even though the advice they gave was valid at that time, their self-image, their confidence, may have been shaken by this new evidence (Mitchell *et al.*, 1992; Thelma, 2000).

The Audit Commission (2001) has categorized change in terms of the scale and style of change. That is, change can be step-change or incremental as well as directive or organic. The scale and style of change will also affect how individuals respond to it. Those involved in practice development activities, therefore, need to be sensitive to the varied reactions that individuals may have to planned change.

CHANGE THEORIES

When considering the process of change, the focus of activity may be on the individual practitioner or a small group of practitioners, or the focus may be on the whole organization or large elements of the organization. There are a number of theories of change which are concerned with achieving change in individuals. These are discussed first, followed by discussion of approaches to change which take a broader perspective, although there is overlap between these two levels of change strategy.

Changing individuals

The classic text, *The Planning of Change* by Bennis *et al.* (1976) was first published over 40 years ago, in 1961. We make no apologies for returning to it now, although some of the language in the book would probably not be used today, as it is a reminder that concern with the process of change has been around for a long time.

Chin and Benne (1976:23) describe three approaches to change: empirical–rational strategies, normative–re-educative strategies, and strategies utilizing some form of power (power-coercive).

The fundamental assumption of empirical–rational strategies is that: '. . . men are rational. Another assumption is that men will follow their rational self-interest once this is revealed to them' (Chin and Benne, 1976:23). Strategies to achieve change using this approach involve providing education for individuals, for example, concerning immunization or overeating: once the individual has understood the message, he is expected to change his behaviour as it is in his self-interest to do so to prevent the diseases caused by not doing so. This approach underpins the diffusion model of dissemination of research findings into practice (discussed below). Once the new knowledge is disseminated, it is expected to lead to change in behaviour due to its power. However: 'The naïve assumption that when research information is made available it is somehow accessed by practitioners, appraised and then applied in practice is now largely discredited' (NHS Centre for Reviews and Dissemination, 1999:2).

The *Effective Health Care* bulletin (NHS Centre for Reviews and Dissemination, 1999) notes that such diffusion or dissemination raises awareness of research findings while research implementation requires action to go further than awareness raising to the application of the findings into practice. Although rationally it may be in a practitioner's best interest to change a particular behaviour, in reality, there are many other factors to take into account. Pringle (1999) found 40 factors, ranging from managerial directives and research findings to control over workload, that influence therapists' everyday practice, demonstrating the complexity of the real world in which practice development takes place.

Normative–re-educative approaches to change are concerned with individuals as members of society and thus acknowledge some of the factors impacting on people which may limit change:

> Changes in patterns of action or practice are, therefore, changes, not alone in the rational informational equipment of men, but at the personal level, in habits and values as well and, at the societal level, changes are in normative structures and in institutionalized roles and relationships.
>
> (Chin and Benne, 1976:23–4)

Change using this approach is concerned with change in the values and beliefs of individuals and in the relationships between individuals in organizations. The introduction of Primary Care Trusts (PCTs) can be seen as a developmental process which requires considerable change in relationships between individuals and organizations. This extensive organizational change requires review of the fundamental beliefs individuals may hold, for example, about leadership of the primary care team, roles of nurses and the place of the consumer in planning services. Primary health care services, according to Meads and Meads (2001), are mediated through a complex network of relationships, and these will be challenged and extended in new ways within PCTs to enable them to become effective primary care organizations. Change, which is going to be seen in practice and in the relationships within and between these new organizations, requires, therefore, changes in the beliefs and values of individuals and the organizations within which they work. Such changes are likely to challenge the self-perception of the individual (Marris, 1986). Approaches to normative–re-educative change include Lewin's model, in which discussion of ideas in groups leads to 'unfreezing' of old ideas and behaviours and then 'moving' and 'refreezing' of new ideas (Lewin, 1952; Benne, 1976; Bryar, 1995; Ewles and Simnett, 1999).

The final approach to change identified above was power–coercive. These strategies use the weight of political, economic or moral power to achieve change, while acknowledging that all approaches to change contain some element of power. The present NHS Plan may be described as a power–coercive approach to change: the Plan has been initiated by the government and mechanisms are in place to monitor and ensure that the plan is implemented (Department of Health, 2000a). As discussed above, this Plan has huge implications for changing the organization and functions of primary health care. We are all participants in this particular change process and have, therefore, experienced the power–coercive approach to change. All of us, and our colleagues, will have our own experiences of this and the other forms of change that will influence our attitudes to the changes involved in new practice development initiatives.

Changing organizations

Arguably, the focus of much change activity in nursing in the past has been on the perceived need to change the individual, and one of the most common approaches to change has been the empirical–rational. However, practitioners in the community do not exist as isolated individuals, but work in partnership with patients/clients and other family members, with other health care practitioners in PCTs and with members of a wide range of organizations, including library staff, housing officers, social workers, lay workers and members of voluntary organizations and many others. The introduction, for example, of joint assessment by district nurses and social services cannot be of greatest benefit to the individuals assessed unless there are far-reaching changes in the working practices within both health and social service organizations (Owens et al., 1995; Department of Health, 2001b).

Action approach to organizations

Several years ago one of the authors was involved in a project that aimed to introduce more individualized care for women into midwifery practice (Bryar, 1995). The main approach to change was through education of midwives to enable them to implement more individualized care in their practice. However, it became apparent that although many midwives were very successful at doing this, others faced constraints that limited the changes that could be made. These constraints related to professional power, hierarchical relationships and lack of autonomy in practice, amongst other things. Silverman (1970) proposed the action approach to organizations which suggests that changes in practice (the action) are dependent on the interrelationship of a number of factors. These include the knowledge held in the wider society about the practice; the attitudes, beliefs and knowledge of the individuals, practitioners and recipients of the practice; and the organizational system within which the practitioners were working. Box 4.1 illustrates the interaction of these three elements on the extent of individualized care experienced by a particular woman from a particular hospital or primary health care team.

By substituting a different issue, for example, home-based rehabilitation after a stroke, the elements that need to be addressed to achieve effective change in each area may be identified.

Systemic change

As indicated in Box 4.1 current practices may be more concerned with meeting the needs of the organization and individuals within that organization than with meeting most effectively the needs of the patient or other members of the community. While the types of change we may be trying to effect in practice development in community nursing may appear to be rather limited, frequently, as Gledhill comments in Chapter 7, they have a wider impact or lead to changes in other areas of the organization. Change in one part of an organization or system will impact on other parts of the system. The action approach to organizations provides one way to look at the interconnections in organizations, and systemic intervention provides another.

The process of systemic intervention identifies the key importance of boundaries in and between organizations and focuses on effecting change at these boundaries (Midgley, 2000). For example, Midgley (2000) and colleagues conducted interviews concerning the process of assessment of older people needing specialist housing. In undertaking these interviews, they identified that the problem lay not so much with

---

Box 4.1 Achieving individualized midwifery care

Society: Knowledge, attitudes, beliefs and values relating to women, pregnancy, family, motherhood, role of midwives, medical power, lay power

$\updownarrow$

Organizational structure: Management systems – hierarchical or collegial; interprofessional relationships; distribution of power in the organization; model of pregnancy held in the organization (i.e. normal in anticipation versus normal in retrospect)

$\updownarrow$

Midwives and women's views: Models of midwifery care and pregnancy they hold; skills including communication and negotiation skills; attitudes towards the role of the midwife

Interaction of these elements =

Individualized personal care giving, increased continuity, choice and control **or**

Impersonal care organized to meet the needs of the organization rather than the woman.

(Bryar, 1995:57)

the process of assessment of housing needs but in the interrelationships between the different agencies involved in utilizing that information. The focus therefore changed from the boundaries between the older people and the assessment process to the boundaries between different groups involved in the use of the assessment information. Work on these areas enabled the development of a shared view of the ideal housing system needed. Thus: '. . . *systemic intervention* is purposeful action by an agent to create change *in relation to reflection on boundaries*' (Midgley, 2000:129).

Another approach to systemic change is that of re-engineering. Re-engineering starts from a concern with the needs of the service user, asking the question: 'How can we reorganize the way we do our work, our business processes, to provide the best quality and the lowest-cost goods and services to the customer?' (Hill and Jones, 2001:487). This approach starts from the needs of the individual person rather than from the functions of staff or the particular attributes of different roles. In the example in Box 4.1, the provision of individualized care by one midwife may be seen as a process of re-engineering this care which had previously been divided between many midwives and other staff. Approaches to integrated nursing, which start from the perspective of the patient in the home rather than from the point of view of the different types of roles held by different nurses in the community, may also be seen as a re-engineering approach to change (Jenkins-Clarke and Carr-Hill, 2001).

DIFFUSION, DISSEMINATION AND IMPLEMENTATION

The definition of practice development (see above) introduced in Chapter 2 suggests that practice development initiatives often involve the development of practice through introduction of new practices based on the findings of research. The different levels within an organization at which change may be needed to achieve a visible change in practice has already been considered; therefore, this section is concerned with methods of change developed to increase the use of research findings

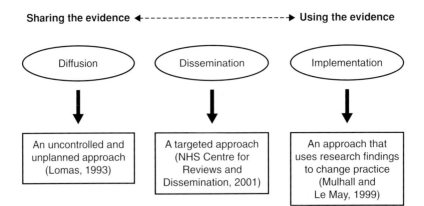

Fig. 4.2 *Research utilization: a spectrum of activity.*

as part of the process of practice development. This process of change is known as 'research utilization'. Research utilization spans a spectrum of activity from sharing the evidence through to using the evidence, with diffusion at one end of the spectrum and implementation at the other (Fig. 4.2). Diffusion, dissemination, implementation are all different aspects of sharing the evidence to bring about a change in practice, and each will be considered in turn.

Diffusion

Diffusion is a passive process (Lomas, 1993) that operates on the assumption that if research findings are published, they will be used. Diffusion begins with the publication of research findings which may or may not be read by nurses in the community. Sometimes an individual will identify a relevant article and this may be pinned to the noticeboard in the practice or health centre; then through a passive process the article is expected to have some influence on practice. However, such an article is unlikely to change practice without an individual being highly motivated and actively promoting the article amongst colleagues and facilitating the change needed. The keyword in relation to the process of diffusion is serendipity (Fig. 4.3): by chance a community nurse reads an article which has relevance to her practice and, if the process of diffusion works, it usually results in awareness raising. It can be seen that this is not a very effective means of achieving improvement in practice.

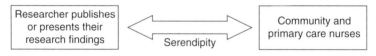

Fig 4.3 *The process of diffusion.*

Dissemination

Dissemination is a more active process (Fig. 4.4) which involves the presentation of research information in accessible formats, such as guidelines, which are then disseminated, following which it is anticipated that they will be used (Lomas, 1993) (*see* Chapters 2, 6 and 7). Ideally the community nurse receives or is alerted to research findings without having to search for them, through a dissemination strategy deployed by the researcher or those who commissioned the research (*see* Chapter 12

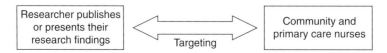

Fig. 4.4 *The process of dissemination.*

for examples of such publications). What actually happens in reality is often limited by resources, including finance and time, and lack of incentive on the part of researchers to actively disseminate their findings.

The key characteristic of dissemination is targeting. Although targeting increases the probability of community nurses receiving research findings relevant to their practice, there is still an element of serendipity. For example, the NHS Centre for Reviews and Dissemination (1997) published an effective health care bulletin on 'Compression therapy for venous leg ulcers'. This was disseminated to key individuals and organizations via a postal distribution list and a series of four conferences in England, Scotland, Wales and Northern Ireland. However, whether individual community nurses received this information will have depended on how it was cascaded in their employing or professional organizations, and whether or not they were one of the few people to attend the conferences. Dissemination, i.e. the targeting of research findings to specific audiences, is also unlikely to change practice, but it may be an important process in bringing research findings to the attention of health care professionals (NHS Centre for Reviews and Dissemination, 1999).

Although the 1991 NHS Research and Development programme invested heavily in the dissemination of research, practice development experience has shown that dissemination on its own is not effective in changing practice. It has been known for some time that: 'the mere provision of information will often fail to accomplish this goal, even when relevant information has been successfully disseminated to an appropriate target audience' (Kanouse and Jacoby, 1988:27). Dissemination of research findings, for example, in the form of guidelines, may be an essential element of research utilization, contributing to awareness raising as a first step in changing in practice. As demonstrated in Chapters 6 and 7, the implementation of guidelines in practice needs active facilitation. Ansell and Watts (2000) in one of the North Thames projects aimed at introducing guidelines in practice, used a number of mechanisms to inform practitioners of the guidelines on the prevention of coronary heart disease, but found that the step from dissemination to change in practice was hard to achieve:

> It had been our hope that most practices would require advice rather than 'hands-on' support to implement the guideline. However, from the experience of the project, time pressure and the scarcity of auditing skills in general practice made this expectation unrealistic in the majority of cases.
>
> (Ansell and Watts, 2000:28)

The processes of diffusion and dissemination may, therefore, be effective to a limited extent in raising awareness of research findings, but implementation of this information requires active support, for example, using the audit cycle (*see* Chapter 2) to achieve change in practice.

The problem with diffusion and dissemination is they are processes built on the assumption that using research findings in practice development is a linear process (Fig. 4.5), but in reality the process is much more complex, as illustrated in Fig. 4.6. In effect, diffusion and dissemination were simple solutions to what is a complex problem. As the journalist H.L. Mencken observed, 'For every complex problem, there is a simple solution, and . . . it's wrong.'

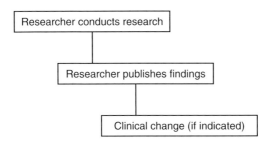

Fig. 4.5 *The linear process of implementation of research findings into practice.*

Implementation

Implementation is an active process of getting research into practice (Fig. 4.7). Implementation, i.e. using research findings in clinical practice, needs to identify the barriers that exist and make use of the interventions most likely to address the barriers (Bury, 1998; *see* Chapter 3). As shown in Box 4.2, there is a whole range of approaches that may be used to support implementation to achieve change in the standards of care, including organizational, individual, managerial and team activities. For implementation to succeed, the process of change management has to be considered and planned.

As indicated in Figs 4.6 and 4.7 and Box 4.2, the process of change is not simply dependent on the quality of the evidence or the structure of the guideline, but is affected by a whole range of factors, including: managerial attitudes, the readiness of the individuals for change and resources to support the change. The need to attend to these factors, and others, is clearly demonstrated in the analysis by Abbott and Hotchkiss (2001) of the failure of their service development project. This project used sound evidence to produce a plan to train a primary care nurse from each of 70 practices to teach pelvic floor exercises to improve urinary continence. In the event, only 16 nurses were trained and few patients, in the required age range, were recruited by the nurses for the pelvic floor education. From the literature, Abbott and Hotchkiss (2001:84, citing Clinical Standards Advisory Group, 1998; Dunning *et al.*, 1998) identify a range of organizational factors that need to be considered when introducing change, including the need to:

- engage GPs;
- work from the bottom upwards;
- be realistic about potential barriers;
- ensure that participants are familiar with the evidence;
- involve patients;
- identify a 'product champion';
- do not try to change primary care in isolation; and
- be incremental.

In their critique of this development project using these criteria, the authors identify many problems, for example, the development process was top-down (*see* Box 4.2) due

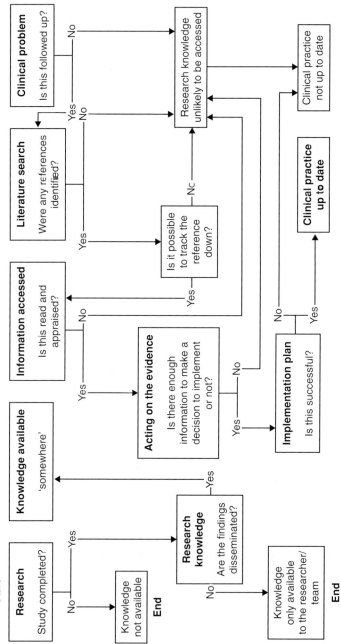
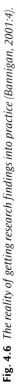

Fig. 4.6 *The reality of getting research findings into practice (Bannigan, 2001:4).*

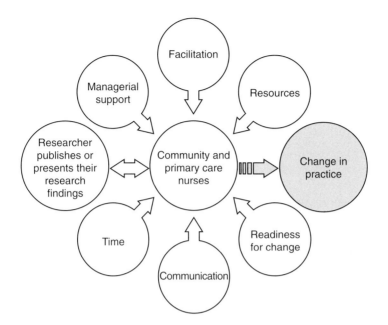

Fig. 4.7 *The complex process of the reality of implementation of research findings into practice.*

Box 4.2 A summary of different approaches to implementation of organizational change

Top-down model ('implementation by control')

- People at the top of an organization incorporate research findings into policy, such as guidelines.
- The expectation is that the change will be incorporated into every aspect of the organization.
- Criticisms of this approach are that it fails to acknowledge how people are and the real world of everyday clinical practice.

Bottom-up model ('implementation as interaction')

- This approach is more laissez-faire, with the aim of minimizing conflict.
- It relies on practitioners to develop strategies for utilizing research findings in their practice settings.

Strategic model ('implementation as evolution')

- It takes a midline between the two previous models, acknowledging that each has insights as well as limitations.
- The focus is the creation of an organizational culture that facilitates learning.

(Adapted from Harrison, 1998)

Table 4.1   *Impediments to a service development concerning pelvic floor education (Abbott and Hotchkiss, 2001)*

Facilitators	Impediments
Engage GPs:	Local Medical Committee and lead GPs not engaged in the project
Work from the bottom upwards	Top-down due to time
Realism about barriers	Length of the assessment; time/costs of release for training not covered;
	GP attitudes to this subject; lack of access to women under 60 with this problem – these and other barriers not anticipated
Familiarity of participants with evidence	Need for more time to examine evidence practitioners were unfamiliar with
Involve patients	Not involved
Use product champion	Continence advisor not in post at start of project
Do not change primary care in isolation	Focus on changing nurses rather than taking a wider primary care perspective
Be incremental	Introduced as a district-wide project

to time constraints imposed by the time available to bid for funds. It was not, therefore, possible to involve the primary care practitioners in the design of the development project, which might have helped them feel more committed to the change process. The difficulties of involving primary care practitioners at the bidding stage are constrained, Abbott and Hotchkiss (2001) suggest, by the fragmented organization of primary care and lack of available time, given the short notice often allowed for project bids to be prepared. Table 4.1 summarizes this and the other factors that inhibited this service development project.

APPROACHES TO CHANGING PRACTICE

Having considered the theoretical underpinnings of change, the different levels at which change may be necessary and the differentiation between diffusion, dissemination and implementation, in this section we are going to consider a number of examples of approaches to change. From these examples, we can draw some principles for effective change. These principles are further demonstrated in Section 2 of this book and are drawn together in Chapter 11. Practice development may operate at the individual, practice/team or organizational level. Iles and Sutherland (2001), in *Organisational Change,* have provided an invaluable resource for all involved in change activities at different levels, reviewing, for example, approaches to organizational level change and identifying and providing the relevant evidence to support the approaches (see Box 4.3). Some of these approaches will be discussed below and others are addressed in Section 2. For example, the rationale and work of a nursing development unit, described in Chapter 10, illustrates a form of group-level change.

The Cochrane Effective Practice and Organization of Care Group is another use-

> **Box 4.3 Approaches to organizational development**
>
> - Organizational-level development, e.g. Total Quality Management.
> - Group-level change, e.g. Self-managed teams.
> - Individual-level change, e.g. through education.
> - Organizational learning and the Learning Organization.
> - Action research.
> - Project management.
>
> (From Iles and Sutherland, 2001)

ful resource for research into interventions to increase research utilization (*see* Chapter 12). They have published an overview of systematic reviews into interventions to increase research utilization (Bero *et al.,* 1998; Thomson, 1998; NHS Centre for Reviews and Dissemination, 1999). They found that written materials or didactic educational meetings have little or no effect. All other interventions were summarized under two headings, strategies with mixed effects (i.e. those where different research studies have shown positive and negative results from similar interventions) and those that have been consistently useful. The mixed evidence of effectiveness led the authors to add the proviso that further research on the relative effectiveness and efficiency of different intervention strategies is required to target such strategies effectively. Strategies with mixed effect include audit and feedback, local opinion leaders, local consensus process and patient-mediated interventions. Educational outreach visits, reminders, multifaceted interventions and interactive educational meetings are strategies that have been shown to be consistently useful. The overriding points to remember are that: (a) just producing written materials or conference papers is not an effective strategy to change practice, and (b) multifaceted, rather than single, interventions targeting different barriers to change are more likely to be effective (NHS Centre for Reviews and Dissemination, 1999; *see* Chapter 3). If people respond differently to change, it is logical that many different strategies will be required to cope with the multiplicity of these different responses.

The marketing approach

All practitioners in the community will be familiar with the approach taken by pharmaceutical and other companies to inform and educate general practitioners, for example, about new drugs, health visitors about new milk products for babies, and district nurses about new continence products. Local representatives of these companies visit individual practitioners in their places of work, where they demonstrate and discuss these products. It must be assumed that this is an effective method of getting the practitioner to adopt the product, and thus change their practice, as thousands of representatives are employed by large multinational companies to undertake this work. If it was not effective, these companies would need to quickly put their resources into other marketing methods.

This was the approach taken in the Framework for Appropriate Care Throughout Sheffield (FACTS) project (Munro, 1995). In this project the aim was to change clinical behaviour to provide evidence-based care in relation to the use of aspirin as a method of secondary prevention; to ensure that a high-quality anticoagulation service was provided for those with atrial fibrillation and that there was an increase in the use of angiotensin-converting enzyme (ACE) inhibitors for those with heart failure. Effective care in these three areas was therefore the 'product' that the team aimed to 'sell' to the practitioners. This process works through individual visits by the project team to the practitioners, and individual discussion of the change process. In this way individuals make up their minds about the product (the change to more effective care). This contrasts, the team suggests, with the more usual approach of seeking consensus or ownership of the process through a group meeting (*see*, for example, Chapters 6 and 8).

The team set this approach within a wider context which takes account of the value placed on the product by practitioners, the credibility of the team bringing about the change, and the need to match the product with the reality of practice. They, therefore, set the marketing approach of working through individuals in the context of a multifaceted approach to change, or in their term 'innovative development', as shown in Box 4.4.

Box 4.4 The FACTS multifaceted approach to change

Three elements of the change process

1. The change programme:
   - Addresses issues of importance to those asked to change;
   - Support provided by key individuals able to take their organizations with them;
   - Multiple interventions tailored to the local situation used;
   - Complements more traditional methods including audit and Continuing Medical Education;
   - Complements contracts and other financial incentives;
   - Motivates individuals by building on their sense of pride.
2. The team promoting change:
   - Has the trust and credibility of those asked to change;
   - Are independent from other organizational agendas.
3. The processes used:
   - Actively translate between different cultures in the NHS;
   - Address the different interests of stakeholders including patients, managers, practitioners;
   - Promote change on the basis of agreement;
   - Actively market the change programme;
   - Watch for resistance and find ways to overcome barriers;
   - Recognize the need to deal with non-rational motivations for change and the importance here of the local context;
   - Integrate the change into the organizational system so that the change is perpetuated;
   - Test out different approaches to innovative development.

(Adapted from Eve *et al.*, 1997:8–10)

Although Eve *et al.* (1997:34) accept that there are 'no magic bullets' to make change happen, they provide a great deal of encouragement to those involved in change processes through their optimism that real change can be achieved through multifaceted approaches:

> The bad news is that there are no magic bullets, no quick-fix tool boxes packed with nifty tricks to achieve this. Instead there is the much more complicated business of listening to people, solving the real world problems they tell you are inhibiting them and inspiring them to change. Multi-faceted programmes built around these principles, tailored to specific purposes, fitted to particular circumstances and purveyed by agencies capable of building trust and credibility are likely to generate real change. In the process such programmes tend to increase both professional satisfaction and the likelihood of future co-operation.

Action research

Action research is an approach to change which incorporates action (i.e. the change process) with research which informs and assesses the impact of the change. It is a form of research that is as concerned with the change process and improvement in services as it is with the conduct of valid, robust research. Hart and Bond (1995) provide a typology of action research, derived from the literature on the subject, showing that the characteristics of action research are that it:

1. is educative;
2. deals with individuals as members of social groups;
3. is problem-focused, context specific and future orientated;
4. involves a change intervention;
5. aims at improvement and involvement;
6. involves a cyclic process in which research, action and evaluation are interlinked;
7. is founded on a research relationship in which those involved are participants in the change process.

(Hart and Bond, 1995:37–8)

Action research was developed by Lewin in the United States of America in the 1940s. Hart and Bond (1995) refer to the description of Kemmis *et al.* (1982) that Lewin's purpose in developing action research was to make use of the experimental process used in social science to tackle some of the major social problems of the time. Action research has, therefore, from the start been seen as a process of development, and, for our purposes here, provides a mechanism to tackle some of the disparities in care provision in the community. The process of action research is described as cyclical involving planning, acting, observing and reflecting (Meyer, 1993). Outside facilitators or an internal facilitator may be involved, but the practitioners and others in the setting are involved in the change process. Hart and Bond (1995) describe a number of different types of action research: experimental, organizational, professionalizing and empowering. These different types give different weight to the seven characteristics above. Two examples, from primary health care, illustrate the different approaches that may be taken using the broad approach of action research to facilitate change in practice. In Box 4.5 a résumé of a project to develop primary health care team-working is given, followed in Box 4.6 by a résumé of the use of a form of action research to gain a better understanding of health visiting.

The example in Box 4.5 demonstrates a number of the criteria of action research identified by Hart and Bond (1995): it is educative, concerned with problem-focused change aimed at improving services in which the different interventions build on each other. This example is broadly based, it involved many practices and addressed a large number of practice/organizational issues. In contrast, the second example is

---

Box 4.5 The Liverpool intervention: using action research to promote change

The Liverpool Primary Health Care Facilitation Project

This project was initially set up in 1989 to help address some of the problems evident at that time in primary care services in Liverpool. It developed through three phases into a large scale action research intervention project. Throughout the three phases the project used participatory methods to help identify with practitioners and others local issues. In phase three, four teams of five people each worked with practices and other organizations '. . . making primary health care facilitation less of a project and more a way of life.' (Thomas and Graver, 1997:179). These teams comprised of primary health care practitioners, for example district nurses, who worked on the project part-time. Five interventions, or 'process parcels' were developed in phases one and two: workshops, road-shows, forums, interactive bulletins and shared projects. These 'process parcels' were used in phase three to identify and help address issues through action cycles of activity, i.e. a process of identification of issues, collection of information/data, development of an intervention, introduction and evaluation of the intervention. Evaluation of action research which takes place in complex settings has also been addressed in this project.

(Thomas and Graver, 1997)

Box 4.6 Using action research to explore health visiting practice

A group of health visitors were concerned about threats to health visiting and used collaborative action research to enable them to explore their practice and describe more adequately what they did as health visitors. A small group was formed and met over a period of eighteen months. During this time they undertook collaborative reflection, a literature search, developed stories about practice and ran an away day for colleagues at which they explored story telling further. Through challenging and gaining a better understanding of the stories the group developed a better understanding of health visiting. Action research enabled them: '. . . to identify concerns, find possible solutions and evaluate and improve practice'.

(Pound et al., 2001:56).

focused on one small group of colleagues. The example is more clearly educational: the focus is to gain greater understanding, but the aim of this understanding is change – to enable more effective practice to be implemented by individual practitioners based on their, and colleagues', better understanding of the complexities of health-visiting practice.

Multifaceted approach to changing organizations

As has been made clear in this section, while individual approaches to change may be very effective, such as the marketing approach, such change methods are more effective when supported by additional levers for change. The NHS Centre for Reviews and Dissemination (1999) report concluded that such multifaceted approaches were more effective in achieving change in practice. The multifaceted approach takes into account the need to ensure that change takes place in the attitudes, behaviours and practice of individuals, in the beliefs and work of teams, and in the structures of organizations, to achieve effective change.

An illustration of this approach is provided by the Teamcare Valleys primary care development project in the South Wales Valleys, funded by the Welsh Office between 1990 and 1993. The remit of the multidisciplinary group appointed to this project was: 'to help develop primary health care in the Valleys area' (Bryar and Bytheway, 1996:13). To this end the project group worked through four approaches: education and training; practical support and advice; communication; and research projects. Education and training activities targeted individuals or groups of individuals in a practice. For example, a study day on immunization was developed for primary health care teams, supported by educational materials and practice reminders. Support and advice were made available to practices through a multidisciplinary group of a GP, nurse and practice manager, who worked with practices on issues concerned with the organization and operation of the practice, for example, recruitment of practice nurses, cervical screening processes and different repeat consultation rates between GPs. Communication activities provided information to practitioners across the 156 practices involved in the initiative and enabled sharing of good practice through activities such as road-shows and a newsletter. Research projects enabled individuals to examine and address an issue in their practice area, such as the meaning of depression to the practice team, women's needs in relation to continuity of community midwifery care, and health behaviours of GPs. Individuals and practices were thus involved in a whole range of activities aimed at encouraging and supporting the development process, and change was evident in the practice of individuals and in the organization of processes within practices. It was concluded that development units seeking wide organizational impact on primary health care need to possess a number of features, shown in Box 4.7.

The South Thames Evidence Based Practice Project (STEP) also illustrates the multifaceted approach to change (McLaren and Ross, 2000; Ross et al., 2001). This project had as its aim the implementation of evidence-based practice in nine NHS trusts. Three change or implementation methods were used: '. . . educational interventions, project (opinion) leaders and clinical guidelines linked to clinical audit' (McLaren and Ross, 2000:101). The project leaders were based in each of the trusts

> **Box 4.7 Requirements for multifaceted primary health care development units**
>
> - Multidisciplinary staff group.
> - Commitment from all stakeholders.
> - A vision of activity shared with stakeholders and practitioners.
> - Secured funding for at least 5 years to enable and demonstrate change.
> - An evaluation strategy from inception of the unit.
> - Flexibility to develop new activities and initiatives.
> - Skills to utilize a wide range of change strategies.
> - Interventions aimed at individuals, practices and the wider primary care organization level.

and led the change process, working with groups in the trust to develop guidelines, undertake audit, develop and provide education on the guideline standards, support implementation and undertake follow-up audit activity. As the evaluation of the complete STEP project shows, change was more likely to occur in those settings in which all partners were likely to benefit. The project utilized a framework to examine the strength of the partnerships underpinning work in each of the trusts. The framework considers the strength of the partnership in six areas: recognition of the need to collaborate on a legitimate basis; assessment of collaborative capacity; purpose of the activity and the ownership of the project; the need to nurture fragile relationships; building trust through principled conduct, and the strength of collaborative pathways (Hudson *et al.,* 1999, cited in Ross *et al.,* 2001). The researchers make the point, similar to Meads and Meads (2001), that considerable effort needs to be put into the development of partnerships to ensure the success of a practice development initiative, in this case, the implementation of evidence-based practice.

PRACTICAL CONSIDERATIONS

While understanding that the theory of change is important, to enable practice development, we also need to pay attention to the practical considerations evinced by the theory. That is, change is difficult, it requires ownership, support, communication and facilitation, and it needs to be focused, project managed and sustainable. The well-known aphorism about genius is apposite for change: change is '1 per cent inspiration and 99 per cent perspiration'. Section 2 focuses on the practicalities of practice development and here we provide a brief commentary on some of the issues.

Change is difficult

The knowledge that change is difficult appears to be known yet constantly overlooked in the planning of change. The discussion (above) of the barriers to research utilization provided an insight into why change is difficult (*see also* Chapter 3). The NHS Centre for Reviews and Dissemination (1999) report suggests that a 'diagnostic analysis' should be used to identify possible issues or barriers. Whatever technique is used, it has to be recognized that for change to be successful these barriers must be overcome. 'Translating ideas into action is (always) tougher than expected' (Audit Commission, 2001:60). Such a realistic approach to change needs to be adopted to ensure it starts and remains manageable.

Focus

Having a focus is one way of keeping a change project manageable. Being focused involves clear prioritization: 'you cannot have ten priorities. If you think you have ten priorities then have you got any priorities?' (Scott, 1992:23).

The UK government's modernization agenda, in its emphasis on the users' experience, provides practice development initiatives with a clear sense of purpose:

> It is only by focusing on user experience that public services can deliver improvements that are relevant and add public value. This means that successful change programmes must begin and end with an understanding of what matters to users.
>
> (Audit Commission, 2001:4)

Developing the focus of the project with all relevant stakeholders also gives those involved a shared sense of purpose. The focus can then be defined explicitly in specific project aims and objectives.

Communication and facilitation

The role of the individual leading the change is critical, as identified by Madhok (1999) early in this chapter. Smith and McClenahan (2000:12), in their evaluation of the North Thames projects to implement guidelines, comment:

> A good project worker is essential. Almost all of the six survey respondents for the primary care guidelines project mentioned the drive, personality, motivation, enthusiasm and/or non-threatening style of the project worker as being a key factor to the project's success. Her genuinely empathetic style helped 'get the trust of the practices', which was in itself a major success.

This means the selection of the person to lead the project is an important decision. This is because the leader will shape the communication and facilitation of the change. Good communication is vital in the fostering of a sense of ownership, so that those involved feel it is as much their project as the project leader's. Facilitation involves translating the original idea into actual practice. Project management is a useful tool to guide the process of turning ideas into action.

Project management

Practice developments are usually one of many things on a community nurse's agenda. This means it is easy to lose sight of an individual project when under pressure. In studies that have analysed why projects are not completed, a weakness identified was in the planning (Bartlett *et al.*, 1997; Caan *et al.*, 1997; Franks, 1998). This type of problem can be avoided by the application of routine project management methods (Usherwood, 1996). Project management, initially developed by the American space programme, is a tool that is widely used in business management and is increasingly used in health and social care (Roberts and Ludvigsen, 1998; Iles and Sutherland, 2001). It is a useful way of monitoring the work related to a project and making sure it is completed. The King's Fund project Promoting Action on Clinical Effectiveness (PACE) found that effective project management was vital to the success of the project (Dopson *et al.*, 1999:10). It is a useful tool in managing change because it provides the 'capacity for managing complex programmes accord-

---

Box 4.8 Approaches to project management

Caan *et al.* (1997) identified four main approaches to project management:

'Do it by the book'

These methods are characterized by detailed protocols, job descriptions related to the project and discipline, i.e. everyone follows everything to the letter.

'Soft analysis'

These methods are a 'collective method of helping the whole team picture where they want to go, and infer routes to attaining that common objective' (Caan *et al.*, 1997:468).

Health service generated approaches – CAPRICODE and PRINCE

CAPRICODE is not recommended for anything other than large-scale projects, such as major capital developments.
PRINCE (Projects in Controlled Environments) is: 'a highly-structured system with a complete set of dedicated documentation in the form of five manuals' (Roberts and Ludvigsen, 1998: 4). Caan *et al.* (1997) describe it as adaptable to small- or large-scale projects. As projects that hope to secure government funding need to adhere to it, training is available on PRINCE (from The Publications Manager, National Computing Centre Ltd, Oxford Road, Manchester M1 7ED, UK).

GANTT charts

Named after the person who invented them. They are horizontal time charts with each stage of the project marked as a line. They are useful because they enable the project team to pictorially represent the timescale of the project and the different tasks involved. A Gantt chart may also be incorporated as an element of the other approaches (above).

ing to a fixed schedule' (Walmsley, 1996:4) and supports successful completion: 'At the start of planning a new project, the adoption of an explicit project management method can help to see the project through to its completion' (Caan *et al.,* 1997:472).

It is important to recognize that project management is more than just time management. All the resources (non-human resources and human relationships), activity and time involved in a project should be considered. Project management also recognizes that things can, and will, go awry. Mechanisms are built into the process to deal with problems as they arise. In short, project management is a means of ensuring that the job gets done. There are different approaches to project management (Box 4.8). Only the generic aspects of project management are outlined here. There are four sets of issues that have to be addressed to manage a project successfully: (1) objectives, outputs and associated quality criteria; (2) time; (3) people and relationships; and (4) non-human resources (Usherwood, 1996). Roberts and Ludvigsen (1998) identify six stages of project management, which are shown in Box 4.9. A word of caution is needed because it is easy to be deceived into believing that project management is a logical, linear process, but the reality is, it is not. The procedures of project management do not have to be implemented rigidly; you have to adapt them to your own situation while still ensuring that you deliver your practice development initiative. The project outcome should always take precedence over process.

A useful introductory text to project management by Roberts and Ludvigsen (1998) provides:

- A toolkit that can be adapted for use in a specific context.
- Case studies of how project management has been used in real-life settings.
- A jargon buster.

Box 4.9 Six stages of project management

- Developing the project idea.
- Assembling the project team.
- Planning the project.
- Making it happen.
- Completing the project.
- Evaluating the project.

(Roberts and Ludvigsen, 1998)

Providing support for change

Many different types of support are required to facilitate successful practice development initiatives from time-out to accessible information sources. A factor cited in several evaluations as a reason for the success or otherwise of an implementation project is management support (Bircumshaw, 1990; Rodgers, 1994; Veeramah, 1995; Humphris *et al.,* 2000). Management support is crucial to the success of practice development projects, because managers often dictate how resources in an organization are used. Richardson and Jerosch-Herold's (1998) appraisal of clinical effectiveness is interesting in this respect because two groups were involved in the change that was being initiated. Managers were educated as well as the senior clinicians, who were perceived as the ones who would actually deliver change. There is recognition in this that those involved in change need support, which means those who provide the support or have control over the environment should be targeted and educated as well.

Sustainability

An important consideration in the development of any change strategy is the extent to which the change will be sustainable after the initial implementation phase. For practice development initiatives to change practice, they have to become the routine practice (*see* Chapter 8). Sustainability may be helped by gaining the initial commitment of all stakeholders, ensuring that the development is supported by research evidence and provides a means of achieving health policy objectives. Through this process a change project may then be developed into a service provided by the particular organization. The development of a community-based rehabilitation service which started as a practice development project and became a funded service provides an illustration of this process.

In 1997–98 the medical director of a health authority was concerned with the lack of equity in access to cardiac rehabilitation for all residents in the health authority area. The cardiac rehabilitation service was based in secondary care and only those people who were motivated or lived near by, had their own transport or access to public transport were able to use the service. The problem was compounded by the large rural geographical area covered by the health authority. One of the team who had developed the Heart Manual (Lewin *et al.*, 1992) worked in the local university. He attended a meeting held with the medical director, which was also attended by one of the authors, who was then the professional lead for health visiting in one of the trusts and also held a joint appointment in the university. A plan was developed to provide a home-based cardiac rehabilitation service for any resident in the health authority area who required it. Stakeholders from the cardiac rehabilitation service, the acute and community trusts, the health authority and practitioners were involved in the development of the project. After presentation of a business case, funding was secured from the health authority for the project and a project lead was appointed along with an administrator. A steering group was established of senior managers from the participating trusts. Health visitors and other practitioners in the community trusts, and ward staff in the acute trusts, were recruited to undertake training in use of the Heart Manual. Funding was provided to enable community practitioners to undertake home visits soon after discharge, at 6 weeks, 6 months and a year post-discharge. Ongoing support meetings and educational events were provided for the community practitioners. Formative and summative evaluation of the service in terms of equity of access, patient satisfaction, levels of physical activity and other factors was undertaken. At the same time the Coronary Heart Disease National Service Framework (Department of

Health, 2000c) was published, providing policy support for community cardiac rehabilitation. At the end of the 2-year project, the steering group concluded that benefits of the scheme were such that the project should continue as part of mainstream service provision, which has happened.

MAKING CHANGE HAPPEN

This chapter has made it clear that getting research into practice is not as simple as choosing an intervention and hoping for the best (Thomson, 1998:7). In changing behaviour a wide range of considerations should be taken into account, including: organizational, economic and community environments, individual beliefs, attitudes and knowledge. If we return to our observation that research utilization is a complex problem with no simple solutions, where does that leave the community nurse with the duty to: 'maintain your professional knowledge and competence' (Nursing and Midwifery Council, 2002:8)? If the current research knowledge is applied to planned change, the chance of success will be increased, although this needs to be done with the proviso that more research is needed for us to understand fully the dynamics of what works and why.

It has already been observed that there is a difference between knowing and doing in relation to change in health and social care; the two are not necessarily coterminous activities. As such, it is important to move from theory to practice, so that we have some understanding of how to apply the theory when involved in practice development initiatives. Obviously it is important to bear in mind what we know about change when planning, conducting and sustaining practice development projects. This knowledge about change could be described or 'guiding principles' for change, i.e. they form the backdrop to your actions when involved in practice development. These principles are shown in Box 4.10.

The publication by the Audit Commission (2001) *Change Here!* is a useful guide to applying what we know about change to the practice development setting. The

---

Box 4.10 Guiding principles for change

- Change is the only certainty.
- Change is challenging.
- People respond differently to change.
- There is a wide range of considerations in planning change.
- Multifaceted interventions are needed.
- Change is a stepwise process in which several barriers have to be removed (Wensing *et al.*, 1998:991).
- Communication is critical to achieving successful change.
- Diligence is needed to achieve sustained change.
- Evaluation is needed to demonstrate that change has taken place.

authors make it clear that although we have a lot of useful knowledge there is no magic formula (Audit Commission, 2001). 'Change initiatives must be "bespoke tailored" by local organisations to tackle the problems facing their communities, if change is to be "owned" locally by the public and by their own staff' (Audit Commission, 2001:4). This means you have to use the guiding principles about change to design a change programme that best fits your practice development initiative and your organization. Unfortunately, 'you cannot simply expect to import someone else's good practice into your own organisation' (Audit Commission, 2001:43).

However, the experience of others can be an extremely useful source of ideas when planning a practice development initiative. Achieving change in the form of initiatives concerned with developing evidence-based practice is the subject of an increasing number of studies. The lessons learnt from two studies have been summarized in Figs 4.8 and 4.9. Figure 4.8 summarizes work that has involved a wide range of health and social care practitioners, whereas Fig. 4.9 summarizes the lessons learnt from nurse practitioners in particular. These summaries indicate that in practice these projects found there was a need to attend to many of the factors that have been discussed throughout this chapter and in the remainder of the book. For example, the need for commitment and support from managers and others; the key role of the facilitator; and the need to identify and address barriers to change.

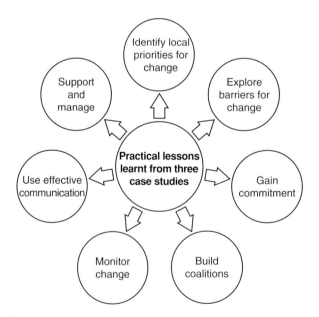

Fig. 4.8 *Learning the lessons 2: Learning from three projects that worked with a wide range of practitioners (from NHS Centre for Reviews and Dissemination, 1999).*

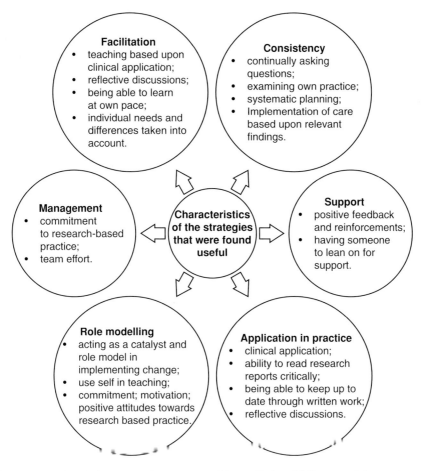

Fig. 4.9 *Learning the lessons 3: What nurse practitioners find useful (from Camiah, 1997).*

Box 4.11 Research utilization projects conducted in the UK

- FACTS (Eve *et al.*, 1997): Framework for Appropriate Care Throughout Sheffield.
- PACE (Dunning *et al.*, 1999): Promoting Action on Clinical Effectiveness.
- CRISP (Caan, 1998): uptake of research findings into clinical practice by the therapy professions.
- NEBPINY (Jones *et al.*, 1996): evidence-based practice in primary care.
- Frontline (Donald, 1997): frontline evidence-based medicine project.
- EPOC: Cochrane Effective Practice and Organization of Care (Effective HealthCare bulletin – Getting evidence into practice); http://www.abdn.ac.uk/public health/hsru/epoc.
- Getting better with the evidence (Wye and McClenahan, 2000): experiences of putting evidence into practice.
- ASPIRE (Hollis and Foy, 2001): Action to Support Practice Implementing Research Evidence; http://www.lancs.ac.uk/users/IHR/ASPIRE.

A number of large-scale projects on evidence-based practice have been conducted in the UK (Box 4.11). There are important lessons to learn from all of these (*see* Chapter 6 for further information on NEBPINY). Taking just one as an example, the lessons from The Promoting Action on Clinical Effectiveness (PACE) project, which involved 16 projects across England covering a variety of clinical topics and a wide range of health care settings, are shown in Fig. 4.10.

APPLYING THE LESSONS LEARNT TO YOUR PRACTICE DEVELOPMENT ACTIVITIES

The PACE project team identified 10 essential tasks for success in practice development (Fig. 4.10). They suggest: 'these tasks need to be managed into a coherent whole with those leading the work having to "link" and "balance" efforts between parallel activities' (Dunning *et al.*, 1999:viii). These tasks can be subdivided into four key activities (Fig. 4.10). Katrina Bannigan has designed a worksheet, using these four activities as headings, as a starting point for those involved in practice development (Fig. 4.11). The Audit Commission publication *Change Here!* is also supported by an interactive web-based tool – www.audit-commission.gov.uk/changehere – and this could also be used to plan change. Remember that whatever tool or information you use to help you plan change, it will have limitations because the author does not know your organization like you do.

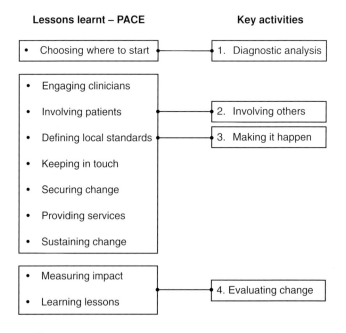

Fig. 4.10 *Lessons from PACE.*

This worksheet can be completed individually or in a group

(1) Diagnostic analysis

Identify barriers to the proposed change/who will be involved/affected by the change/facilitators of change (e.g. skills and resources)?

Choose the focus for your practice development activity and where to start.

(2) Involving others

Which clinicians and patients need to be involved? How could you facilitate their involvement?

Fig. 4.11 *Brainstorm ideas for planning your practice development.*

(3) Making it happen

Define local standards using knowledge of relevant research/Outline methods for keeping in touch/securing change/providing services/sustaining change.

(4) Evaluating change

Monitoring and evaluating change – How are you going to measure impact? How will you share the lessons learnt?

Use these notes as a basis for developing your approach to change in your practice development. This worksheet can be revisited during the process.

Fig. 4.11 *continued.*

CONCLUSION

In this chapter we have sought to give an overview of the process of change. We have discussed theoretical approaches to change and provided examples of change applied to practice from our own and others' experiences. The processes and principles of change discussed here are further illustrated in Section 2. As this chapter demonstrates, there are considerable resources available to provide help with planning practice development activities. Many of the examples we have included make the point that practice development is challenging and we may not have emphasized the positive aspects of the process enough. The process of change presents huge rewards in terms of the learning achieved by individuals, their sudden insights and the development of teamwork engendered by the process. Equally, it can lead to improvements in care and the satisfaction of knowing that, for example, a consistently high quality of service is being provided to everyone with a venous leg ulcer. As discussed in Chapter 1, the advent of PCTs provides practitioners with a real opportunity to influence and lead real change, which has the potential to improve the quality of clinical care. Change can lead to a reallocation of resources and better use of practitioners' time. The above may all be positive experiences or outcomes of the process of change involved in practice development and may provide elements of the evaluation of the development. As indicated in Chapter 2 our approach to change and practice development includes a need to incorporate evaluation into the change process. This has not been discussed in this chapter but is the subject of Chapter 5.

REFERENCES

Abbott S and Hotchkiss J 2001 It takes more than clinical effectiveness to change nursing practice: an unsuccessful project in the nurse promotion of urinary continence. *Clinical Effectiveness in Nursing* 5: 81–7.

Ansell M and Watts C 2000 Promoting the secondary prevention of coronary heart disease through clinical guidelines in primary care in Barking and Havering. In: Evans D and Haines A (Eds) *Implementing Evidence-Based Changes in Healthcare.* Radcliffe Medical Press, Abingdon, pp. 17–37.

Audit Commission 2001 *Change Here! Managing Change to Improve Local Services.* Audit Commission, London.

Bannigan K 2001 Annual AOTMH Lecture 2001: 2001 Sharing the evidence for mental health occupational therapy practice. *Mental Health OT* 6(2): 4–9.

Bartlett H, Ersser S, Davies C and Chappell S 1997 Characteristics and dissemination of nursing research in an acute healthcare trust. *NT Research* 2(6): 414–22.

Benne KD 1976 The process of re-education: An assessment of Kurt Lewin's views. In: Bennis WG, Benne KD, Chin R and Corey KE (Eds) *The Planning of Change,* 3rd edn. Holt, Rinehart and Winston, New York, pp. 315–27.

Bennis WG, Benne KD, Chin R and Corey KE (Eds) 1976 *The Planning of Change,* 3rd edn. Holt, Rinehart and Winston, New York.

Bero LA, Grilli R, Grimshaw JM, Harvey E, Oxman A and Thomson MA 1998 Closing the gap between research and practice: an overview of systematic reviews of interventions to promote the implementation of research findings. *British Medical Journal* 317: 465–8.

Bircumshaw D 1990 The utilisation of research findings in clinical nursing practice. *Journal of Advanced Nursing* 15: 1272–80.

Bryar RM 1995 *Theory for Midwifery Practice.* Palgrave, Basingstoke.

Bryar RM 1999 Using research in community nursing. In: McIntosh J (Ed.) *Research Issues in Community Nursing.* Macmillan, Basingstoke, pp. 6–28.

Bryar R and Bytheway B (Eds) 1996 *Changing Primary Health Care. The Teamcare Valleys Experience.* Blackwell Science, Oxford.

Bury T 1998 Getting research into practice: changing behaviour In: Bury T and Mead J (Eds) *Evidence Based Healthcare: A Practical Guide For Therapists.* Butterworth-Heinnemann, Oxford.

Caan W 1998 *Uptake of Research Findings into Clinical Practice by the Therapy Professions.* Report for the NHS Executive North Thames R&D Directorate, London.

Caan W, Wright J and Hampton-Matthews S 1997 Start as you mean to go on; Project management for beginners. *Journal of Mental Health* 6(5): 467–72.

Camiah S 1997 Utilisation of nursing research in practice and application strategies to raise research awareness amongst nurse practitioners: a model for success. *Journal of Advanced Nursing* 26: 1193–202.

Chambers 1994 *The Chambers Dictionary.* Chambers Harrop Publishers Ltd, Edinburgh.

Chin R and Benne KD 1976 General strategies for effecting change in human systems. In: Bennis WG, Benne KD, Chin R and Corey KE (Eds) *The Planning of Change,* 3rd edn. Holt, Rinehart and Winston, New York, pp. 22–45.

Clinical Standards Advisory Group 1998 *Report on Clinical Effectiveness, Using Stroke Care as an Example.* HSC 1998/108. The Stationery Office, London.

Department of Health 2000a *The NHS Plan.* Department of Health, London.

Department of Health 2000b *Towards a Strategy for Nursing Research and Development.* Proposals for Action. Department of Health, London.

Department of Health 2000c *National Service Framework Coronary Heart Disease. Modern Standards and Service Models.* Department of Health, London.

Department of Health 2001a *Shifting the Balance of Power within the NHS – Securing Delivery.* Department of Health, London.

Department of Health 2001b *National Service Framework for Older People. Modern Standards and Service Models.* Department of Health, London

Donald A 1997 Front-line evidence based medicine project: report to the implementation committee. North Thames RHA, London.

Dopson S, Gabbay J, Locock L and Chambers D 1999 *Evaluation of the PACE Programme: Final Report.* Oxford Healthcare Management Institute, Templeton College, Oxford University, Oxford.

Dunning M, Abi-Aad G, Gilbert S and Livett H 1998 *Turning Evidence into Everyday Practice.* King's Fund, London.

Dunning M, Abi-Aad G, Gilbert D, Hutton H and Brown C 1999 *Experience, Evidence and Everyday Practice Creating Systems for Delivering Effective Health Care.* King's Fund, London.

Evans D and Haines A (Eds) 2000 *Implementing Evidence-based Changes in Healthcare.* Radcliffe Medical Press, Abingdon.

Eve R, Golton I, Hodgkin P, Munro J and Musson G 1997 *Learning from FACTS Lessons from the*

Framework for Appropriate Care Throughout Sheffield (FACTS) Project. ScHARR Occasional paper 97/3. ScHARR, University of Sheffield, Sheffield.

Ewles L and Simnett I 1999 *Promoting Health. A Practical Guide.* Bailliere Tindall in association with the Royal College of Nursing, Edinburgh.

Franks A 1998 Managing research and development. In: Baker M and Kirk S (Eds) *Research and Development for the NHS: Evidence, Evaluation and Effectiveness,* 2nd edn. Radcliffe Medical Press, Abingdon, pp. 127–40.

Greenhalgh T (2001) *How to Read a Paper: The Basics of Evidence Based Medicine.* BMJ Publishing Group, London.

Harrison S 1998 Implementing the results of research and development in clinical and managerial practice. In: Baker MR and Kirk S (Eds) *Research and Development for the NHS: Evidence, Evaluation and Effectiveness.* Radcliffe Medical Press Ltd, Abingdon.

Hart E and Bond M 1995 *Action Research for Health and Social Care. A Guide to Practice.* Open University Press, Buckingham.

Heywood P 2000 The changing nature of service provision. In: Tovey P (Ed.) *Contemporary Primary Care. The Challenges of Change.* Open University Press, Buckingham, pp. 26–42.

Hill CWL and Jones GR 2001 *Strategic Management Theory,* 5th edn. Houghton Mifflin Company, Boston.

Hollis S and Foy R 2001 *ASPIRE Action to Support Practice Implementing Research Evidence.* Lancaster University, Lancaster.

House of Lords: Select Committee on Science and Technology 1988 *Medical Research and the NHS Reforms.* HMSO, London.

Hudson B, Hardy B, Henwood M *et al.* 1999 In pursuit of inter-agency collaboration in the public sector. *Public Management* 1(2): 235–60.

Humphris D, Littlejohns P, Victor C, O'Halloran P and Peacock J 2000 Implementing evidence based practice: factors that influence the use of research evidence by occupational therapists. *British Journal of Occupational Therapy* 63(11): 516–22.

Iles V and Sutherland K 2001 *Organisational Change. A Review for Healthcare Managers, Professionals and Researchers.* National Co-ordinating Centre for NHS Service Delivery and Organisation R&D, London School of Hygiene and Tropical Medicine, London.

Jenkins-Clarke S and Carr-Hill R 2001 Changes, challenges and choices for the primary health care workforce: looking to the future. *Journal of Advanced Nursing* 34(6): 842–9.

Jones K, Wilson A, Russell I, Roberts A, O'Keefe C, McAvoy B, Hutchinson A, Dowell A and Benech I 1996 Evidence-based practice in primary care. *British Journal of Community Nursing* 1: 276–80.

Kanouse DE, Jacoby I (1988) When does information change practitioners' behavior? *International Journal of Technology Assessment in Health Care* 4: 27–33.

Kemmis S *et al.* 1982 *The Action Research Reader,* 2nd edn. Deakin University Press, Australia.

Lewin K 1952 Group decision and social change. In: Swanson GE, Newcomb TM and Hartley EL (Eds) *Readings in Social Psychology,* Revised Edition. Henry Holt and Company, New York, pp. 459–73.

Lewin B, Robertson IH, Cay EL, Irving JB and Campbell M 1992 A self-help post MI package – The Heart Manual effects on psychological adjustment, hospitalisation and GP consultation. *Lancet* 339: 1036–40.

Lomas J 1993 Diffusion, dissemination and implementation: who should do what? *Annals of New York Academy of Sciences* 703: 226–35.

Madhok R (1999) Getting research into practice: a case study. *Journal of Public Health Medicine* 21: 3–7.

Marris P 1986 *Loss and Change.* Routledge and Kegan Paul, London.

McLaren SMG and Ross F 2000 Implementation of evidence in practice settings: some methodological issues arising from the South Thames Evidence Based Practice Project. *Clinical Effectiveness in Nursing* 4: 99–108.

Meads G and Meads T 2001 *Trust in Experience. Transferable learning for primary care trusts.* Radcliffe Medical Press, Abingdon.

Mencken HL *www.io.com/gibbonsb/mencken* (accessed on 28 March 2001).

Meyer JE 1993 New paradigm research in practice: the trials and tribulations of action research. *Journal of Advanced Nursing* 18: 1066–72.

Midgley G 2000 *Systemic Intervention: Philosophy, Methodology, and Practice.* Kluwer Academic/Plenum Publishers, New York.

Mitchell EA, Taylor BJ, Ford RP, Stewart AW, Becroft DM, Thompson JM, Scragg R, Hassall IB, Barry DM, Allen EM *et al.* 1992 Four modifiable and other major risk factors for cot death: the New Zealand study. *Journal of Paediatric Child Health* 28 (Suppl. 1): S3–8.

Mulhall A and Le May A (Eds) 1999 *Nursing Research Dissemination and Implementation.* Churchill Livingstone, Edinburgh.

Munro J 1995 Facing the FACTS *Health Service Journal* **105**(5473); 5 October: 26–7.

NHS Centre for Reviews and Dissemination 1997 Compression therapy for venous leg ulcers. *Effective Health Care* 3(4).

NHS Centre for Reviews and Dissemination 1999 Getting Evidence into Practice. *Effective Health Care* 5(1) .

NHS Centre for Reviews and Dissemination 2001 Available at http://www.york.ac.uk/inst/crd/dissinfo.htm (accessed on 26 March 2001).

NHS Executive 1998 *Achieving Effective Practice: A Clinical Effectiveness and Research Information Pack for Nurses, Midwives and Health Visitors.* Department of Health, Leeds.

Nursing and Midwifery Council 2002 *Code of Professional Conduct.* Nursing and Midwifery Council, London.

Owens P, Carrier J and Horder J (Eds) 1995 *Interprofessional Issues in Community and Primary Health Care.* Macmillan Press Ltd, Basingstoke.

Pound R, Dams M, Gammon K, Martindale J, Page C and Stapleton J 2001 Practice and knowledge: an approach to action research. *Community Practitioner* 74(2): 54–7.

Pringle E 1999 *Examining the Research-practice Gap in the Therapy Professions.* University of Kent, Canterbury, Kent.

Richardson B and Jerosch-Herold C 1998 Appraisal of clinical effectiveness – an ACE approach to promoting evidence-based therapy *Journal of Clinical Effectiveness* 3(4): 146–50.

Roberts K and Ludvigsen C 1998 *Project Management for Health Care Professionals* Butterworth-Heinemann, Oxford.

Rodgers S 1994 An exploratory study of research utilisation by nurses in general medical and surgical wards. *Journal of Advanced Nursing* 20: 904–11.

Ross F, McLaren S, Redfern S and Warwick C 2001 Partnerships for changing practice: Lessons from the South Thames Evidence-based Practice project (STEP). *NT Research* 6(3): 817–28.

Scott M (1992) *Time Management.* BCA, London.

Silverman D 1970 *The Theory of Organisations.* Heinemann, London.

Smith L and McClenahan J 2000 Evaluation of the Purchaser-led Implementation Programme.

In: Evans D and Haines A (Eds) *Implementing Evidence-based Changes in Healthcare.* Radcliffe Medical Press, Abingdon, pp. 1–16.

Thelma A 2000 Breath Easy. *Health Service Journal* 110(5703): 1.

Thomas P and Graver L 1997 The Liverpool intervention to promote teamwork in general practice: an action research approach. In: Pearson P and Spencer J (Eds) *Promoting Teamwork in Primary Care. A Research-based Approach.* Arnold, London, pp. 174–91.

Thomson MA 1998 Closing the gap between nursing research and practice. *Evidence-Based Nursing* 1(1): 7–8.

Tovey P (Ed.) 2000 *Contemporary Primary Care. The Challenges of Change.* Open University Press, Buckingham.

Usherwood T 1996 *Introduction to Project Management in Health Research a Guide for New Researchers.* Open University Press, Buckingham.

Veeramah V 1995 A study to identify the attitudes and needs of qualified staff concerning the use of research findings in clinical practice within mental health care settings. *Journal of Advanced Nursing* 22(5): 855–61.

Walmsley, S 1996 Project Management as a tool in implementing major organisational change: a case study. *Local Government Policy Making* 23(1): 3–12.

Wensing M, Van Der Weijen T, Grol R 1998 Implementing guidelines and innovations in general practice: which interventions are effective? *British Journal of General Practice* 48: 991–7.

Wye L and McClenahan J 2000 *Getting Better with Evidence.* King's Fund, London.

5

Evaluating developments in practice

Jane Griffiths, Andrew Leeming and Rosamund Bryar

Purpose of this chapter

- To define evaluation.
- To consider the place of evaluation in practice development.
- To consider different approaches to evaluation.
- To outline methods used to undertake evaluation.

INTRODUCTION

In Chapter 2 practice development was defined thus: 'Development [is] work directed towards introducing an innovation or the improvement of a service or process, often based on the findings of research' (NHS Executive, 1998:6). Practice development in community nursing is, therefore, essentially about bringing about change in some aspect of the service provided by community nurses. The impact of that change should be felt potentially by any or all of the following: patients and other service users, carers, staff, other social and health care organizations. The collection of information to assess the impact of the innovation or change provides the evaluation of the practice development initiative.

The need to evaluate health service interventions has been brought to the fore by the importance that is now placed on efficiency within the NHS, but it is not just the incentive to save money that has highlighted the importance of establishing whether practices are successful or otherwise. A key component of both evidence-based practice and clinical effectiveness is evaluation of the intervention. For developments in practice to occur, it is imperative that at the end of the project, and in many cases throughout the project, successes and failures are scrutinized so that best practice is continued. In fact Russell (1996:4), in his definition of development, implies that a developmental process can only be said to have been undertaken when implementation and evaluation of that implementation are undertaken together:

> Development is the *experimental* introduction into practice of alternative clinical procedures or methods of care, together with the *simultaneous evaluation* of their effectiveness, efficiency or both. This includes health technology assessment, Phase III drug trials, and other pragmatic trials designed to choose between alternatives in clinical practice. It excludes service developments that are not subject to evaluation. [*our emphases*].

There is perhaps limited sense in carrying out a project if we do not enter it with at least some idea about what we aim to achieve and how we will establish whether this has occurred (*see* Chapters 4 and 8).

Evaluation is a familiar concept to community nurses, as it is a component of the nursing process. It is not always something that is carried out particularly well, however, partly because it can sometimes be difficult to establish outcome measures against which to gauge success. Perceived difficulties in carrying out evaluation and a reluctance to subject a project to scrutiny, particularly if it did not go according to plan, are reasons that community nurses may avoid evaluating developments in practice. The intention of this chapter is to dispel any fears that you may have about evaluation and to demonstrate that it is an invaluable and indispensable component of developing practice in community nursing.

WHAT IS EVALUATION?

Evaluation is about assessing the success of an intervention against a set of criteria. Such comparison, as Ovretveit (1998:13) notes, enables: '. . . people to make better informed practical decisions'. The history of evaluation shows that for over 100 years efforts have been made to refine and develop the process of evaluation. Guba and Lincoln (1989) describe this development in terms of generations, each building on and developing the evaluation process.

The first generation of evaluators were concerned with measurement, for example, the measurement of the scores of children in school tests. The second generation of evaluators were concerned with description and introduced the possibility of formative not just summative evaluation, i.e. evaluation while the project was in progress not just when it was complete (see below). Objectives were set, for example, for educational programmes and evaluation provided descriptions of the extent to which the objectives of the programme were met. The next phase of the development of evaluation, described by Guba and Lincoln (1989) as the third generation, was when the value judgements implicit in evaluation were made explicit. Evaluators were asked to make judgements about the totality of a programme, including, for example, the relevance of the goals set for the programme, in addition to the extent to which the goals were met. Fourth-generation evaluation, which Guba and Lincoln (1989:50) describe as the coming of age of evaluation, is characterized by its focus on: '. . . the claims, concerns, and issues of stakeholders . . .' in the process of the evaluation. The fourth-generation evaluation process starts from a position of involvement of stakeholders, as opposed to the position of earlier approaches which distanced stakeholders from the 'objective evaluator'. However, Guba and Lincoln (1989) make the important point that, as in a multigeneration family, several generations may coexist together. So, for example, current schemes for testing children at different ages in schools could be described as being first- or second-generation approaches to evaluation. A fourth-generation approach to such testing would take into account stakeholders, such as the local community, parents, the local authority and others, to devise a process of evaluation which might more accurately describe the achievements of these children, in this school, in the context of their community.

The focus and outcome of the process of evaluation is on the practical, on making an assessment of the achievements of the new development against criteria identifying what it was planned to achieve. St. Leger and Walsworth-Bell (1999:116) provide the following definition of evaluation in the context of health services, stating that evaluation is: 'The critical assessment, on as objective a basis as possible, of the degree to which entire services or their component parts (e.g. diagnostic tests, treatments, caring procedures) fulfil stated goals.'

An example of the evaluation of two leg ulcer clinics may help to illustrate this process, as shown in Box 5.1.

Box 5.1 Aim of service development: to prevent the recurrence of leg ulcers

It was the practice at the local leg ulcer clinic to refer patients back to their own district or practice nurse once the leg ulcer was healed. Evidence suggests that recurrence is lowest in those people who use Class 3 hosiery but that there may be problems for patients in applying this hosiery. To reduce the rate of recurrence, all those with healed ulcers were reviewed on a regular basis at the leg ulcer clinic. In practice this led to the clinic becoming overloaded, and a separate clinic was started for people with healed leg ulcers. An evaluation of the impact of the healed leg ulcer clinic was undertaken to assess whether the clinic was having an impact on the rate of recurrence and whether reassessment of patients' Doppler readings was taking place. Although the total patients in this study are only 32, seen over a three year period, the evaluation showed that: 'The percentages of recurrence fell from 50% in 1997 to 16% in 1999 . . .' and: 'In 1998, 42% had one follow-up Doppler assessment and in 1999, 66% had at least two follow-up Doppler assessments, thus demonstrating an improvement in safety and quality of care' (Bentley, 2001:140).

WHY DO WE NEED TO EVALUATE PRACTICE DEVELOPMENT ACTIVITIES?

The suggestion that practice development initiatives should be subjected to systematic examination may not be greeted with universal agreement from community nursing colleagues, and the question of why such evaluation should take place and what are the benefits of evaluation needs to be addressed. Ewles and Simnett (1999:88) suggest that those undertaking evaluation need to have thought through their reasons for the evaluation: 'You need to be clear about why you are evaluating your work, because this will affect the way you do it and the amount of effort you put into it'.

There are many reasons to evaluate, and a 'quick think' with colleagues will throw up a whole host of reasons. Some of the more obvious ones would include:

- ensuring that the activities are having the desired effect;
- minimizing waste of resources;
- improving materials and methods;
- assessing the validity of scepticism about the effectiveness of an intervention;
- assessing whether activities are ethical;
- improving local practice;
- spreading good practice;
- giving local professionals and other actors within a project the satisfaction of knowing how useful or effective their work has been;
- unearthing unplanned benefits.

Some colleagues may be sceptical of the benefits of evaluation, seeing it merely as a means for managers and other decision makers to appear to be basing their decisions on a sound basis. Evaluation may be just another panacea for uncertainty which, as Pawson and Tilley (1997:xii) suggest: '. . . could go the way of shamanism; it could be a philosophical kingdom without a court; it could turn out to have a shelf life of the typical agony aunt; it could be heading for a fall'.

Others may argue against the apparent constant need for evaluation of interventions which have been shown in many different settings to be effective (Nutbeam, 1998). Nutbeam, for example, draws attention to the large number of evaluations of health promotion interventions that have taken place and argues that evaluation is not always necessary when an intervention which has been shown to be effective is introduced into a new setting. The counter argument to this is that evidence from practice development activities and from some researchers (Pawson and Tilley, 1997) shows that the context within which the developmental activity is taking place is crucial to its success. So that even though an intervention may have been shown to be effective in many different settings, in a particular context it may be unsuccessful due to a problem in the new setting. Therefore, even though an intervention may have demonstrated its value on many occasions, we also need to recognize that an intervention does not simply exist in a vacuum and that any outcomes will be dependent on other factors particular to the new context.

Another reason that people may not be enthusiastic about evaluation is because, to a greater or lesser degree, it involves making a judgement about the worth of the intervention. This is not a new issue. Barnsley et al. (1986:7) described the problem:

> . . . evaluation is generally considered to be an unpleasant process. It is a process of making judgements, but that is something we all do everyday. The difficulty is that the term 'evaluation' implies criticism and a 'them' and 'us' situation. Evaluation has traditionally been a process in which someone, often a funding agency or its agent, stands apart from the group and passes judgement on its success or failure.

Wass (1994:94) sees evaluation as very value laden: 'a process by which we judge the value or worth of something'. Hawe (1994) further suggests that it also reveals 'what' is valued about an intervention and what is not. Dixon and Sindall (1994) and Everitt (1995) agree that evaluation is a judgement-passing activity. As indicated at the beginning of this chapter, evaluation is clearly about making judgements about a development activity: such judgements help to demonstrate the positive benefits of the development as well as indicating areas which may require further attention.

FORMATIVE AND SUMMATIVE EVALUATION

Evaluations can take place either *formatively* or *summatively*. Formative evaluation is carried out throughout the project and informs the project's development. It therefore aims to affect the outcome of the project. Summative evaluation occurs at the end of the project to establish whether the aims of the project have been met. Waks and Barak (1996) define this difference as follows:

> Summative evaluation carried out at the end of program implementation tends to rely on defined evaluation designs and uses publicly accepted instruments which have established reliability and validity and reflect the concerns of the sponsor or decision makers.

> (Waks and Barak (1996:171)

and

> Formative evaluation aims to improve a program while it is still in process, when development and implementation of materials and techniques is still taking place. It provides feedback to both learners and teachers about success and failure in mastering specific areas of knowledge or skills.

> (Waks and Barak 1996:172)

Summative evaluation may therefore use 'harder' quantitative measures, such as audit, questionnaires or patient satisfaction surveys. Formative evaluation may use qualitative techniques such as informal interviews and focus groups to inform the direction of the project.

TOOLS FOR EVALUATION

As is the case when conducting a research study, the key issue in evaluation is to use the right tools for the job. For most researchers the debate about whether to employ quantitative or qualitative methods has been replaced by recognition of the importance of using the best technique to answer the research question (*see* Chapter 3). Quantitative and qualitative methods are therefore often combined to best effect. The same is true of evaluation. Certain developments in community nursing practice are best evaluated using quantitative methods. The healing rate of a leg ulcer can be measured, for example, as can the recurrence rate of leg ulcers in the practice population (*see* Chapter 6). Other changes, such as a health promotion initiative or a community-based programme, may be better evaluated using mainly qualitative approaches, that is asking the various participants about their experience of the development, using, perhaps, conversational-style interviews (*see* Chapter 9).

There are many methods that can be used when conducting an evaluation, but before we look at these, it is important to consider the different approaches to evaluation.

TYPES OF EVALUATION

There are a number of ways to classify the different approaches to evaluation. Ovretveit (1998) describes four perspectives or approaches to evaluation: the developmental, experimental, economic and managerial. In practice, these approaches are not necessarily separate, for example, a developmental evaluation may include aspects of economic and managerial evaluation. Following a brief overview of experimental, economic and managerial approaches here, we are going to focus on developmental evaluation, including the evaluation of community development projects. Developmental evaluation is the approach to evaluation most commonly used by community nurses in practice development, as illustrated by the examples in Section 2 of this book.

Experimental evaluation

Experimental evaluation is based on the principles of experimental research. In the laboratory situation it is possible to select an experimental and a control group and to apply an intervention, for example, a treatment or drug to the experimental group. By measurement of the differences between the control group and the experimental group at the end of the experiment, it is possible to state the impact or effectiveness of the intervention. Undertaking such research in the real world is more difficult as those of you who have been involved in studies of, for example, new drugs or new dressings, will be aware (*see*, for example, Chapter 6, in which use of an experimental design in the evaluation of the implementation of guidelines is described).

To overcome some of these problems quasi-experimental designs have been devised (Cook and Campbell, 1979; Campbell and Stanley, 1963). These designs aim to take into account aspects of the real world, such as the difficulties of randomly allocating people to control groups (*see* Chapter 8) or preventing people telling each other about treatments they are having or even, as is a common experience in community nursing, sharing prescribed drugs! All these actions will undermine the true experiment.

Experimental evaluation can be used to evaluate practice development activities, and Box 5.2 provides an illustration of such an evaluation (Griffiths and Evans, 1995). This study concerns the impact of a nursing-led in-patient service and is included here as many of the factors measured are of importance to community nurses receiving these patients back into the community.

Pawson and Tilley (1997) provide a detailed critique of experimental evaluation

---

Box 5.2 Experimental evaluation of a nursing-led in-patient service

This study is concerned with the impact of the service on patient outcomes and has an hypothesis which is tested through the collection of data about patients on the experimental ward and the control ward.

Null hypothesis*: Admission to the nursing-led ward will result in patient outcomes which are no different from those achieved through current services.

Results showed that this hypothesis was not supported in relation to a number of the outcomes. Patients on the experimental ward experienced:

Reduced length of stay in acute beds

Lower psychological distress

Higher proportion discharged to their own home/sheltered accommodation

Lower incidence of chest infections and pressure sores

(Griffiths and Evans, 1995:7,39)

*Null hypothesis: The hypothesis that states that there is no relationship between the variables under study (Polit and Hungler, 1991:650)

---

with its focus on the outcomes, rather than the processes and context into which the change is introduced. They argue that the focus for evaluation should be on the context and the processes within that context which actually facilitate the change: that these processes are more important than the actual outcomes, as without them change will not occur (*see* Chapter 4). They suggest two guiding principles for real istic research (in evaluation) (Box 5.3).

Thinking about our own experiences of practice development and the introduction of change in practice, we are all aware of the importance of the context, the support given by key individuals and the receptiveness of clients on the effectiveness of the development. For example, clinical supervision may be welcomed by one group of

---

Box 5.3 Realistic evaluation

Axiom 1
Research [evaluation] has to answer the questions: what are the mechanisms for change triggered by a programme and how do they counteract the existing social processes?

Axiom 2
Research [evaluation] has to answer the questions: what are the social and cultural conditions necessary for change mechanisms to operate and how are they distributed within and between programme contexts?

(Pawson and Tilley, 1997:75,77)

Box 5.4 The Promoting Action on Clinical Effectiveness (PACE) programme

This programme focuses on organisational development to secure the implementation of evidence for a specific clinical condition.

Lessons concerning the need to be aware of the context in which the change will take place

Be clear about what needs to change

Link the work into local priorities

Consider the options available for securing change

Understand local issues and potential barriers to change

Take into account the needs and interests of GPs and primary health care teams.

(Dunning *et al.,* 1998:1,59,60)

---

community nurses who are able to access education, decide the best approach for their group and are given permission by managers to use work time in this developmental activity. Another group may reject clinical supervision when the context within which it is introduced is punitive, education available to staff is limited and recording systems rather than the actual activity of clinical supervision are given priority. The value of the practice development initiative of clinical supervision in both cases is the same, but the outcomes in terms of more effective practice, better supported and informed staff (for example) are very different, due to the different contexts. As shown in Box 5.4, the need for awareness of the local context is one of the lessons from the interim, or formative, evaluation of the PACE programme (Dunning *et al.,* 1998) (*see also* Chapter 4).

Experience has shown that detailed preparation is essential to lay the ground for effective work with primary care. It is easy to be tempted to develop a plan of action that assumes that all practices are broadly the same. Such an approach is likely to fail. It is essential to recognize and build on the diversity of primary care. Practices will have their own interests and pressures – and it is unrealistic to expect them all to go forward at the same rate. They are each likely to have their own agenda and will raise different interests in debates about clinical effectiveness. This diversity may limit the use of experimental evaluation in practice development in community nursing. However, quasi-experimental designs such as cohort studies, discussed in Chapter 8, may offer more potential.

Economic evaluation

The focus in economic evaluation is on the costs of a particular activity: the resources used and the outcomes achieved. An additional aspect of economic evaluation is an assessment of the costs incurred by not using the available resources to provide other services. This assessment acknowledges that resources are limited, and providing resources for one activity of necessity limits resources for other activities, i.e. there is an opportunity cost to any planned activity (Ovretveit, 1998) (*see* Chapters 8 and 10).

An example of an economic evaluation is found in an evaluation of a Community Rehabilitation Team (Luker *et al.*, 1999). The team was established to allow the early discharge home of patients following an acute in-patient episode necessitated by, for example, a fall or a stroke. The Community Rehabilitation Team (CRT) was a team of physiotherapists, occupational therapists and nurses who were able to provide rehabilitation in the home that would otherwise have been carried out in hospital. The CRT was one of a series of initiatives that had been set up to provide 'intermediate care services' in the home that would be normally offered in hospital.

Various methods were used to carry out the evaluation. Patients and carers were interviewed to explore their perceptions of the new service. Members of the CRT were interviewed to capture their views, as were the Rehabilitation Assessment Teams in the hospitals who discharged the patients to their homes. An economic evaluation also took place as it was important to establish whether the service was cost-effective. The patients were required to keep diaries to record the expenses that they had incurred during the period of rehabilitation at home. Also, the cost per in-patient day was compared with the cost of sending the CRT to the patient's home for the period of rehabilitation, which was usually less than 6 weeks.

The result of the evaluation indicated that patients did not incur any extra cost as a result of receiving their rehabilitation at home. Although it was difficult to interpret the data as there were so many factors to take into account, it appeared that it was no more expensive, and perhaps cheaper, to rehabilitate patients in the home. These findings must, of course, be viewed in relation to the benefits to patients. The patients preferred to receive rehabilitation at home and appeared to do better in this setting than the artificial environment of the hospital.

Economic evaluation is an important aspect of evaluation that must be considered in the preparation of evaluation of any new development. The Wanless Report (Wanless, 2002) provides emphasis to the importance of economic issues or fundamental to the development of the health service.

Managerial evaluation

Ovretveit (1998) describes managerial evaluation as an approach to evaluation which developed during the last decades of the twentieth century. The managerial perspective on evaluation:

> . . . views health interventions from the point of view of health service funding bodies, health managers and their concerns and tasks. In general the management perspective is concerned with two things: ensuring that things are done properly, and trying to use available resources to the best effect.
>
> Ovretveit, 1998:137.

Such evaluations may be undertaken by the managers themselves but they are frequently undertaken by an outside organization, consultants or inspection bodies, for example. The teams that are undertaking the work for the Commission for Health Improvement (CHI) provide an example of the managerial approach to evaluation.

Another example is provided by the work of the Audit Commission, which illustrates, in its statement of purpose, the principles of the managerial perspective on

---

Box 5.5 Evaluation findings in *First Assessment*

District nurses provide most of the professional nursing care given to patients who live at home. But trusts face a rising demand for these services at a time when large numbers of district nurses are nearing retirement and fewer are qualifying. Given these pressures, trusts need to review the ways in which they organise, manage and deliver district nursing services.

Issues addressed: demand for district nursing services; quality of services using leg ulcer and continence care as examples; cost of district nursing services; and the future role of the district nursing services.

The findings of the evaluation identified a number of areas needing development, including:

- The lack of a clear service definition
- Mismatch between resources and patients' needs
- Unwarranted variations in the quality of clinical performance

The evaluation report recommended to managers that: 'In order to improve the quality and efficiency of district nursing, managers need to. . . address 14 areas,' including:

- Influence and manage demand by improving the referral process
- Invest in professional development programmes for community nursing staff to support the development of self-managing teams
- Appoint team facilitator(s) to provide continuing support to teams

(Audit Commission, 1999:5, 18–19, 95, 112)

---

evaluation: 'The Audit Commission promotes the best use of public money by ensuring the proper stewardship of public finances and by helping those responsible for public services to achieve economy, efficiency and effectiveness' (Audit Commission, 1999:cover). The managerial approach to audit is illustrated in Box 5.5, which outlines some of the issues addressed by the Audit Commission in its report: *First Assessment*, an evaluation of the district nursing service (Audit Commission, 1999).

Managerial evaluation is, therefore, more concerned with issues of effectiveness and value at the level of the service or organization. If the outcomes of interest to managerial evaluation illustrated in Box 5.5 are compared with the outcomes examined in experimental evaluation (*see* Box 5.2), the differences in the focus of these two different approaches to evaluation are apparent.

Developmental evaluation

Developmental evaluation has as its focus the more immediate implementation of change as part of the process of evaluation than the other approaches described above. While approaches to developmental evaluation using, for example, case study design, may not have change as part of the design, developmental evaluation and change are frequently considered as part of an interrelated process (Ovretveit, 1998). Given the value judgements that are always embedded in evaluation, though not always acknowledged (Ong, 1993), participatory approaches to evaluation may be more acceptable to those who are part of the service being evaluated.

Developmental evaluation may be undertaken by those in the practice situation or by outside evaluators. Examples of this approach to evaluation include methods such as reflection on practice, where individuals in the setting undertake the evaluation; action research approaches, where those in the setting may undertake the evaluation themselves or may undertake the evaluation with outside researchers; and other forms of social research, such as case study, in which those in the setting participate but the evaluation is led by outside researchers.

Nurses are very familiar with the process of reflection and the utilization of reflection in clinical supervision as an aid to change (*see* Chapter 7). Action research has become a more widely used approach to research in nursing over recent years. Action research involves assessment, implementation of change and evaluation of the change process (*see* Chapter 8). The participants in the service being evaluated using an action research approach may be more or less involved in the process of evaluation and change (Hart and Bond, 1995).

Case study approaches to evaluation use a variety of methods to collect information from the range of different people involved in, or affected by, the practice development initiative (Bryar, 2000). Information is also collected regarding the context in which the development is taking place. For example, a case study approach was used to evaluate the impact of the introduction of two different nurse practitioner service models (Holden *et al.*, 2000). Data were collected from patients, the practice teams and a wider range of stakeholders using one-to-one and group interviews, focus groups, questionnaires, video recordings and analysis of records. By collecting a wide range of information, the aim is to provide a more complete picture of the impact of the development on all those involved rather than just presenting the evaluation from the perspective of one group.

One type of service evaluation which requires the involvement of those involved in the setting in the evaluation is the evaluation of community development initiatives. Health visitors, community midwives, school nurses and other nurses working in the community are increasingly involved in community development initiatives as part of their public health work. Community development is an open-ended process, with community development professionals and other practitioners often taking a less prominent role in driving the objectives/focus of activity. This begs the question: 'Who is driving the need for outcome measures?' As with all types of service evaluation, different stakeholders are involved. Freeman *et al.* (1997) acknowledge that the range of stakeholders involved in the evaluation of community development work, such as community-orientated public health, will have different interests. Purchasers will be interested in value for money and outcomes; participants will be concerned to identify new activities and professionals will be concerned to learn about the effectiveness of methods being used (Freeman *et al.*, 1997:87). Evaluation and community development may seem rather incompatible, but where community development is being funded by external bodies it is often a necessity, as well as being of help to those participating in the activity. Participatory research methods are considered to be the most appropriate approach to monitoring and evaluation of such developments (Noponen, 1997).

Perhaps the most common problem with evaluation of community development is finding an appropriate form of measurement with which all can agree. This problem will now be addressed in some detail.

Much community development work is by 'character' invisible, a simple causal chain which links a health-promoting activity with a change in health status has long been discredited. Even by asking the apparently simple question: 'What would the outcome have been if the activity had not taken place?' a large number of complex issues are raised. It soon becomes clear that even where clear benchmarks or baselines can be identified, this is insufficient because it assumes that they remain static and that all subsequent changes are caused by the activity alone. Outcome measures within community development are difficult to clarify; this in part is because community development:

- Is an emergent process.
- Is very open ended and has a broad and shifting focus.
- Intentionally the framework takes a wide perspective on health and outcomes.
- Tries to address things that apparently cannot be changed.
- It is difficult to specify the appropriate time scale or level.

Luck and Jesson (1995) would add that evaluation of community development is made all the more difficult because community development is:

- relatively new and
- relatively unconventional,

and within community development projects:

- most objectives and priorities change, because events are in a continuing process (outcomes rarely match objectives);
- there are few tangible, measurable outcomes (it is difficult to measure changes in behaviour which will have long-term effects);
- there is no control group.

So how do we know whether our objectives have been achieved? Freeman *et al.* (1997) suggest that there is a need within the evaluation to measure both processes and outcomes. In their description of criteria which define success, Hawe *et al.* (1995:114) identify these two elements: '. . . linked with changes in the community itself, its networks, its structures, the way in which people perceive the community, ownership of community issues, perceived and actual "empowerment" in health and social issues'. They go on to state what they believe must be measured, including: how residents value 'community'; how well local people articulate their views; how active they are in contributing to the achievement of community goals and how well they manage and accommodate conflict of differences.

Flecknoe and McLellan (1994:13) offer three key questions to gauge success, which fit well with the above views: (1) Have local people been involved in the identification of needs? (2) Have local residents taken a lead in the development of the activities? (3) Have local people's skills of participation in and leadership of activities been strengthened? Within community development projects Everitt (1995:63) contends that evaluation becomes: 'the process concerned with providing opportunities for conversations to take place amongst those involved in the project'.

Measuring success is made all the more difficult because of the frequent inability to link an intervention to an outcome (Ashton and Seymour, 1990; Downie *et al.*, 1994; Naidoo and Wills, 1994; DeFriese and Crossland, 1995; Dixon, 1995). Community development is, by its very nature, a long-term process, and this also has implications when looking at success. Flecknoe and McLellan (1994:13) note that:

> Superficially impressive results can be achieved quickly but only by rejecting the vital long-haul approach of slowly building up relationships and confidence in favour of opportunistic, funding-led developments and/or the establishment of groups run directly by paid staff rather than local residents.

Freeman *et al.* (1997) suggest that, in relation to community-orientated primary care, outcomes may be linked to processes through looking at outcome effects on primary care services; other agencies; on health and on communities. They stress the need for participants to generate their own outcome measures.

Lessons from the challenges of evaluation of community development work may be applied to other service developments in community nursing. So, for example, in district nursing certain outcomes are difficult to measure, such as which components to address when developing a service for carers of people with dementia. Yet, clearly, throughout a project such as this, it would be important to make a judgement about what is most and least helpful, in order to develop the project in the right direction. Through adopting the participatory approach to evaluation used in community development, evaluation would involve those with dementia, carers, health professionals and others. These people would all contribute to the evaluation design, identify the aspects of process and outcomes to be investigated and participate in the generation and analysis of the data.

METHODS FOR EVALUATION

Perhaps the best way to consider the methods that can be used for evaluation is to look at examples of developments in practice from the field and consider how these could be evaluated. This should help to de-mystify the process and give you some practical ideas to apply to your practice. There are many methods available to you when you carry out an evaluation (Box 5.6). The aim is to find the most sensible tools for the job, in other words, the method that is likely to give you the most accurate and helpful results. This is similar to conducting a research study (Parahoo, 1997). Many of you will have taken part in a research study and have been asked something by questionnaire that is almost impossible to answer but would have been more appropriately asked during an interview, when you could have clarified questions and expanded on your answers. There may have been other times when you would have preferred the anonymity of a questionnaire to a face-to-face interview. You are the experts in your field of practice. You know what a sensible, workable approach to eliciting information would be, because you know what would be a reasonable question to be asked yourselves. You may need to be quite imaginative when devising appropriate ways to obtain the information that you require.

Consider a development in practice that involved setting up a community leg ulcer clinic as an alternative to treating patients in their own homes. Reasons for

---

Box 5.6 Examples of methods for collecting information for evaluation

- Questionnaires
- Interviews
- Document analysis
- Record analysis
- Observation
- Literature reviews
- Physiological measurements
- Focus groups

---

setting up the clinic may include improving leg ulcer management by standardizing practice and reducing cost. In other words, increasing efficiency and clinical effectiveness in leg ulcer management. So how might you evaluate whether this has happened?

You would probably be interested in comparing healing rates with patients nursed in their own homes, so you may be looking at the number of weeks it takes to heal the ulcer. You may be interested in looking at rates of recurrence of leg ulcers over a fairly long period of time, a year or more (*see* example in Box 5.1). This quantitative, i.e. numerical, information could be collected using a separate recording sheet or by examination of nursing records.

You may wish to compare treatment protocols at the clinic with recorded treatment protocols in care plans in the home and compare these to clinical guidelines for leg ulcer management. This information, which would be both quantitative, for example, how frequently were the guidelines followed, and qualitative, for example, what evidence was there in the records for deviation of care from the guidelines, could be obtained by content analysis of the nursing records.

You may decide to carry out a patient satisfaction survey or to interview patients about their views of the service, to ensure that it meets their needs as well as yours. A survey would require the development of a questionnaire collecting quantitative and qualitative information, while an interview schedule, which would be more or less structured, would be needed for the interviews.

You would probably compare the cost of the service in terms of nursing time and dressings over the period of treatment. To obtain this information you would need to collect data from nursing records of activities, and additional financial data.

From this example, it can be seen that evaluation of many nursing interventions requires the use of both quantitative and qualitative methods to elicit the information needed to make a judgement about the success of a practice development initiative.

The leg ulcer clinic is an hypothetical example. The next example is from practice where audit was used to bring about change (Griffiths and Hutchings, 1999). Audit is a cyclical process in which an initial (baseline) audit is carried out to assess the extent to which an area of practice deviates from ideal practice, which would preferably be evidence-based. A development in practice is implemented to bring actual practice closer to ideal practice. Practice is re-audited and further developments are introduced if necessary. Thus, practice is developed, re-audited, developed, re-audited and so on, cyclically, so that it incrementally becomes closer to ideal practice. This is similar to formative evaluation.

In Griffiths and Hutchings' practice as district nurses it was noted that the evaluation part of the nursing process was rarely carried out well, if at all. They decided to conduct a baseline audit of care plans to discover the extent of the problem. They looked at three areas of care and developed evidence-based standards with which to compare recorded practice. The three areas were leg ulcer care, bath care and catheter care. They also looked at the way in which the care plans were organized, such as the sequence of documentation and the amount of crossing out on the care plans. As a result of the initial audit, various developments were introduced to address identified problems, for example, training was offered in catheter care, leg ulcer care and care planning. The care plans were then re-audited a year later to see whether there was any improvement, which in some areas there was. Table 5.1 shows the data for leg ulcer management, which indicates an improvement over the year. There was, however, scope for further development in all areas of recording of leg ulcer data, so the cycle of practice development continued.

When using audit to evaluate an area of care, the methods available are very similar to the methods that are used by researchers (Closs and Cheater, 1996). Whichever method will get the best information is the method that should be used. If, for example, you were interested in auditing the uptake of a clinical guideline, you would be interested in assessing the extent to which practice had changed. You might look at documentation such as care plans or you might observe practice; you might interview patients or issue a questionnaire to staff. You may do all of these, and anything else that seemed relevant when assessing change within the particular area of practice. The wide range of approaches to such evaluation are demonstrated in Evans and Haines (2000) collection of approaches to the introduction of evidence-based change including the use of guidelines. Marshall, in Chapter 6, illustrates both qualitative outcomes and quantitative change that was achieved through the facilitated introduction of guidelines in the NEBPINY (Network for Evidence-Based Practice in Northern and Yorkshire) project. Quantitative findings from the same project using an audit of records are provided in Rolfe (2001), demonstrating the value of audit to highlight areas requiring further development as well as areas in which improvements have been made.

The examples so far have been of summative evaluations. So what about formative evaluations that inform the course of the development? If, for example, you were

Table 5.1 *Evaluation of use of care plans using audit: leg ulcer data (number of care plans, n = 26)*

	Recorded in initial audit	Recorded in re-audit
Measurement	9	15
Assess wound edges	4	5
Assess wound bed	14	14
Level of exudate	13	6
Colour	2	2
Skin condition	9	12

setting up a journal club to introduce evidence-based practice and to develop critical thinking skills, you might be interested in evaluating the club early on in its development, to ensure that members were obtaining maximum benefit from it. You would possibly look at attendance rates and you may interview group members to ask them how the journal club was affecting the way that they practised. You may issue a short questionnaire. As attendance is entirely voluntary, you would probably not want to do anything threatening, such as testing participants' critical appraisal skills or observing their practice to see whether it was evidence based! A focus group interview may be an appropriate approach, where group members share ideas about the future direction of the journal club meetings.

To summarize this section, the methods used in any evaluation must be appropriate to the aspect of the practice development activity that is being evaluated. Certain methods will be more appropriate for experimental, economic, managerial or developmental evaluation, but none are limited to use for a particular type of approach to evaluation.

WHOSE CRITERIA SHOULD BE USED IN EVALUATION?

An important consideration when carrying out an evaluation is: whose criteria should be used to make a judgement about success or otherwise? Think about the way in which community nursing services are evaluated by purchasers, in terms of numbers of patient contacts. How relevant is the number of patients/clients that a community nurse visits? How about the content of those visits? In the early 1990s the Audit Commission carried out an evaluation of the district nursing service (Value for Money Unit, 1992). As a result of shadowing G- and H-grade district nurses in three community trusts in England, they concluded that the skill mix in district nursing teams was too rich, and that much of the work of the district nursing sister could be carried out by staff nurses who, at that time, did not hold a district nursing qualification. The report recommended reducing the number of G- and H-grade district nurses by a half (Value for Money Unit, 1992). District nurses across the country were concerned by the way in which their work had been reduced to a series of tasks, and the tasks assigned to less-qualified staff. They felt that the subtler, qualitative elements of their work had been missed by the Audit Commission. It is often much more difficult to quantify the less measurable components of a development in practice, but it may be quite meaningless to reduce it to something that is outwardly more manageable.

The issue of who should actually evaluate a project is controversial. It is apparent that the views of everyone involved in a project must be taken into account, as illustrated in Chapter 9. Everitt (1996:174) suggests that: 'The ways in which practice is talked about, and communicated, by those in it, users, workers, funders, managers, policy-makers, differ'. Forss and Carlsson (1997:498) in their essay 'The quest for quality – or can evaluation findings be trusted?' found: 'Evaluations of high quality were almost always the result of team work. Seldom did a lone evaluator produce a "good" or "excellent" report, but lone evaluators produced most of those that were "inadequate". Russell and Willinsky (1997) would concur and cite Barrack and Cogliano (1993:37) to emphasize the point: '. . . crucial to successful program evalu-

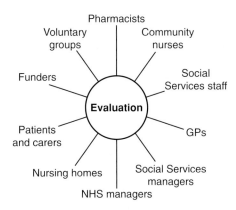

Fig. 5.1 *Potential stakeholders involved in an evaluation of a new community nursing service.*

ation is the involvement of the stakeholder' and 'The challenge is to create a situation where the various stakeholders are actually listening to each other' (Barrack and Cogliano, 1993:90). However, there is a note of caution from Noponen (1997:31): '. . . the reality does not always measure up to the ideal, however, and many techniques, touted as participatory, still essentially "extract" information from participants, however creatively they do it'.

It is apparent that the production of 'many truths' through 'many voices', while being seen as 'best practice', throws up numerous dilemmas. Everitt (1996:187) describes the situation as:

> . . . who should be the judges? Clearly, it is inappropriate for evaluators alone to make judgements about the value of practice — their task is to contribute to the generation of evidence and to facilitate the process of judgement-making informed by the evidence. Equally, it is not appropriate for practitioners alone to be judges of their own practice . . . .

For anyone embarking on evaluation of a service development perhaps the most important thing is to identify and take into account the views of all the stakeholders involved (Fig. 5.1). As discussed in Chapter 4, the involvement of stakeholders in the change/practice development is vital to its success and they should therefore already be involved in the process, enabling their participation in the evaluation process.

FINDING 'TRUTH' IN EVALUATION

When carrying out an evaluation and choosing the most appropriate method, it is important to be aware of the interests of those involved in the evaluation and how these might affect the honesty of the responses you are seeking. We must be aware of the power that certain parties hold over different groups of people. This is more than simply not choosing a particular group to participate in an evaluation. It is about acknowledging the power dynamics within an evaluation; for example, a group may take part in an evaluation, but the answers they give to the questions asked are those that they know the interviewers want to hear. This could be due to any number of circumstances: they want the project to appear good/useful, fear of money/funding being taken away, not wanting to look like they have failed, not wishing to 'rock the boat' or simply being unaware of the purpose of the evaluation. Drewett (1997:191) illustrates these dilemmas in relation to evaluation of services for mental health users:

> ... mental health users' expectations may be shaped by the funding situation nationally and locally of services, so that they may be unlikely to express negative attitudes towards their own services because of concerns about possible closures; their disability may hinder their desire to speak publicly or privately for fear of stigma and exclusion; they may lack information about their rights and also what is available and, depending on their own social and political background, users may have divergent views about the responsibility of the state and their families to provide different services. All these factors may affect the extent to which certain methods work with different client groups or situations.

From the above we can see that when user views are taken into account, caution is advised. We also need to be aware of how user opinions will be viewed and observed by others. The issue is particularly relevant when we consider how 'institutions' have, in the past, viewed lay knowledge, seeing it as inferior to professional expertise, with lay knowledge relegated to the status of the personal and subjective and the professional elevated to the heights of 'expert' (*see* Chapter 3). Wynne (1994) examines this issue in relation to the public understanding of science, where public rejection or resistance to a scientific development is interpreted as a lack, amongst members of the public, of adequate technical knowledge to enable them to come to the 'correct' understanding: 'Thus, when publics resist or ignore a program advanced in the name of science, the cause is assumed to be their misunderstanding of the science' (Wynne, 1994:362). Rather such rejection may be based on the different world views or models held by members of the public, which may have as much validity as the models of the so-called 'experts'. Naturally we must also remember that people like to be nice! 'Being nice' can mean communication can get 'blocked', people refrain from plain criticism or avoid any language or statements that may trouble participating parties.

Involvement of users in all forms of research and evaluation is becoming much more usual (Hanley, 2001). However, participation is not straightforward. While we can rightly articulate that those who are affected by a policy initiative are often the people who know the problems and how to act upon them, in practice it is difficult to involve them in evaluation. There are important practical issues as well, such as tracing project participants. Groups and other participants may have moved on since their period of involvement, with some groups having a higher turnover of participants than others (Brooks *et al.*, 1997).

CONCLUSION

To summarize, therefore, although evaluation is by no means straightforward, especially when attempts are being made to quantify the unquantifiable, it is vital that attempts are made to overcome potential difficulties and that evaluations are carried out. Practice development initiatives should not be rushed into without consideration of what the project is trying to achieve and how success or otherwise will be established. There are many controversial issues to be addressed in the field of evaluation, not least who should be evaluating the project. The most relevant person or group to carry out the evaluation will depend upon the nature of the project itself. So, for example, if we are evaluating a community leg ulcer clinic, it may be appropriate for a managerial-style evaluation to take place that looks at, amongst other things, the cost effectiveness of the service. If, however, we are evaluating a community development initiative, in which members of the public have been involved throughout, then it is important that their voices are heard in the evaluation of the project. Equally, if the project is about development of the community, the evaluation should take place throughout the project in order to inform its course. With the evaluation of a leg ulcer clinic it may be more appropriate to collect a sizeable database of healing rates, cost, etc. before drawing conclusions about the way ahead. As we have argued here, involvement of all stakeholders will result in a more rounded evaluation reflecting different perspectives and concerns.

The most important point to consider when working out how to evaluate a project is to take the approach and use the methods that best fit the purpose of the project. In this sense evaluation is similar to research. There are no universal right or wrong ways to conduct the process, just the most appropriate method for the project. Evaluation is not something that should be feared. It need not be complicated and should facilitate, rather than hinder, the course of a project, because a clear idea about what is to be achieved can only help the project to run more smoothly and help the transfer of projects into mainstream services.

REFERENCES

Ashton J and Seymour H 1990 *The New Public Health. The Liverpool Experience.* Open University Press, Milton Keynes.

Audit Commission 1999 *First Assessment. A Review of District Nursing Services in England and Wales.* Audit Commission, London.

Barnsley J, Ellis D and Jacobson H 1986 *An Evaluation Guide for Women's Groups.* Women's Research Centre, Vancouver.

Barrack C and Cogliano J 1993 Stakeholder involvement: Mythology or methodology? *Evaluation Practice* 14(1): 33–7.

Bentley J 2001 Preventing unnecessary suffering: an audit of a leg ulcer clinic. *British Journal of Community Nursing* 6(3): 136–44.

Brooks F *et al.* 1997 *Heart of Our City Project – Final Evaluation Report.* Sheffield Hallam University/University of Sheffield/Health Research Institute/Medical Care Research Unit.

Bryar R 2000 An examination of case study research. *Nurse Researcher* 7(2): 61–78.

Campbell D and Stanley J 1963 *Experimental and Quasi-experimental Evaluations in Social Research.* Rand McNally, Chicago.

Closs SJ and Cheater FM 1996 Audit or Research: what is the difference? *Journal of Clinical Nursing* 5(4): 249–56.

Cook TD and Campbell DT 1979 *Quasi-Experimentation*. Rand McNally, Chicago.

DeFriese G H and Crossland C L 1995 Strategies, guidelines, policies and standards: the search for direction in community health promotion. *Health Promotion International* 10(1): 69–74.

Dixon J 1995 Community stories and indicators for evaluating community development. *Community Development Journal* 30(4): 327–36.

Dixon J and Sindall C 1994 Applying logics of change to the evaluation of community development in health promotion. *Health Promotion International* 9(4): 297–309.

Downie R S, Fyfe C and Tannahill A 1994 *Health Promotion: Models and Values*. Oxford University Press, Oxford.

Drewett A 1997 Evaluation and consultation. Learning the lessons of user involvement. *Evaluation* 3(2): 189–204.

Dunning M, Abi-Aad G, Gilbert D, Gillam S and Livett H 1998 *Turning Evidence into Everyday Practice*. King's Fund, London.

Evans D and Haines A (Eds) 2000 *Implementing Evidence-based Changes in Healthcare*. Radcliffe Medical Press, Abingdon.

Everitt A 1996 Values and evidence in evaluating community health projects. *Critical Public Health* 6(3): 56–65.

Ewles L and Simnett I 1999 *Promoting Health. A Practical Guide,* 4th edn. Baillière Tindall, Edinburgh.

Flecknoe C and McLellan N 1994 *The What, Why and How of Neighbourhood Community Development*. Community Matters, London.

Forss K and Carlsson J 1997 The quest for quality – or can evaluation findings be trusted? *Evaluation* 3(4): 481–501.

Freeman R, Gillam S, Sherrin C and Pratt J 1997 *Community Development and Involvement in Primary Care. A Guide to Involving the Community in COPC*. King's Fund, London.

Griffiths JM and Hutchings W 1999 The wider implications of an audit of care plan documentation. *Journal of Clinical Nursing* 8: 57–65.

Griffiths P and Evans A 1995 *Evaluation of a Nursing-led In-patient Service: An Interim Report*. King's Fund, London.

Guba EG and Lincoln Y 1989 *Fourth Generation Evaluation*. SAGE Publications, Newbury Park.

Hanley B 2001 Taking on the Policy Research Programme. *Consumers in NHS Research Support Unit News* Summer: 1

Hart E and Bond M 1995 *Action Research for the Health and Social Care, a Guide to Practice*. Open University Press, Buckingham.

Hawe P 1994 Capturing the meaning of 'community' in community intervention evaluation: some contributions from community psychology. *Health Promotion International* 9(3): 199–210.

Hawe P, Degeling D and Hall J 1995 *Evaluating Health Promotion*. Maclennan and Petty, London.

Holden J, Bryar R and Campion P 2000 *An Evaluation of Two Models of Nurse Practitioner Development*. Final Report. Centre for Community Nursing/Department of Public Health and Primary Care, University of Hull, Hull.

Luck M and Jesson J 1995 *Community Health Development Evaluation – Public Sector Management Research Centre*. Aston Business School, Birmingham.

Luker K, Waters K, Austin L, Griffiths J and Gosden T 1999 An evaluation of the South Manchester community rehabilitation project. Unpublished report, University of Manchester, Manchester.

Naidoo J and Wills J 1994 *Health Promotion. Foundations for Practice.* Baillière Tindall, London.

National Health Service Executive 1998 *Achieving Effective Practice: A Clinical Effectiveness and Research Information Pack for Nurses, Midwives and Health Visitors.* Department of Health, Leeds.

Noponen H 1997 Participatory monitoring and evaluation – a prototype internal learning system for livelihood and micro-credit programs. *Community Development Journal* 32(1): 30–49.

Nutbeam D 1998 Evaluation of health promotion – progress, problems and solutions. *Health Promotion International* 13(1): 27–44.

Ong BN 1993 *The Practice of Health Services Research.* Chapman & Hall, London.

Ovretveit J 1998 *Evaluating Health Interventions.* Open University Press, Buckingham.

Parahoo K 1997 *Nursing Research. Principles, Process and Issues.* Macmillan, London.

Pawson R and Tilley N 1997 *Realistic Evaluation.* SAGE Publications, London.

Polit DF and Hungler BP 1991 *Nursing Research.* JB Lippincott Company, Philadelphia Pennsylvania.

Rolfe MK 2001 The NEBPINY programme (Phase 1). Changing practice – testing a facilitated evidence-based programme of primary care. *The Journal of Clinical Governance* 9: 21–6.

Russell I 1996 What is research and development? *Refocus: The NHSE Northern and Yorkshire Research and Development Newsletter.* Issue 4 Spring: 4–5.

Russell N and Willinsky J 1997 Fourth generation educational evaluation: the impact of a post-modern paradigm on school based evaluation. *Studies in Educational Evaluation* 23(3): 187–99.

St. Leger AS and Walsworth-Bell JP 1999 *Change-promoting Research for Health Services.* Open University Press, Buckingham.

Value for Money Unit (1992) *The Nursing Skill Mix in the District Nursing Service.* HMSO, London.

Waks S and Barak M 1996 Role of evaluation in an interdisciplinary educational program. *Studies in Educational Evaluation* 22(2): 171–9.

Wanless D 2002 *Securing Our Future Health: Taking a Long-Term View.* Final Report. HM Treasury, London. http://www.hm-treasury.gov.uk/consultations_and_legislation/wanless/consult_wanless_final.cfm (accessed on 9 December 2002)

Wass A 1994 *Promoting Health. The Primary Health Care Approach.* WB Saunders Baillière Tindall, Harcourt Brace and Company, London.

Wynne B 1994 Public understanding of science. In: Jasonoff S, Markle G, Petersen J and Pinch T (Eds) *Handbook of Science and Technology Studies.* SAGE Publications, London, pp. 361–88.

Section 2

In this section five approaches to practice development are presented, illustrating and building upon the chapters in Section 1:

- The use of audit and guidelines introduced using a process of practice facilitation.
- The introduction of guidelines supported by clinical supervision.
- An action research approach involving a wide multidisciplinary team.
- Participatory appraisal to identify what change is actually needed within a community.
- The approach of a Nursing Development Unit.

Each example is presented by someone involved in the process of development and provides, as well as the description of the process, an analysis of the lessons learnt and what might have been done differently.

Each of the chapters gives a practice example which serves to illustrate the underlying principles presented in Section 1: the need for clear definition of terms and the practice development initiative; consideration of the evidence underpinning the change process; awareness of the multifaceted nature of the change process and consideration of the different forms of evaluation open to those involved in practice development.

Lessons from the chapters in Section 2 are brought together in Section 3 of the book, in Chapter 11, with information from Section 1 to provide a template of issues which need to be considered as we embark on practice development activities.

6

Implementation of evidence-based guidelines in primary care: The NEBPINY experience

Joyce L. Marshall

Purpose of this chapter

- To review the literature on the use of guidelines in practice.
- To demonstrate the process of guideline implementation in primary care.
- To identify the importance of the change context on guideline implementation.

INTRODUCTION

In this chapter some of the advantages and problems associated with the use of evidence-based guidelines for the care of patients with venous leg ulcers in primary care are discussed, emphasizing the importance of the context within which the guidelines are to be implemented. The literature on the use of guidelines to disseminate research evidence is reviewed to provide the current theory on guideline implementation. Two case studies of practices participating in a research project evaluating the use of guidelines are presented to illustrate how differently primary care teams tackle the same problem given the same resources. As the facilitator of the process of guideline implementation in these practices, I present my interpretation of some of the key issues relevant to the use of evidence-based guidelines. Discussion of these and some of the results from other practices taking part in the research study enable me to present the principles that may be of use to any community practitioner attempting to improve quality of care in the community setting.

A REVIEW OF THE LITERATURE

The need for evidence-based practice

There has been growing interest in recent years in the application of the principles of evidence-based practice, which has been defined as the: 'conscientious, explicit and judicious use of current best evidence in making decisions about the care of individual patients' (Sackett *et al.*, 1996:2) (*see* Chapter 3). Evidence of considerable variation in practice, both across different regions of the UK and in different countries, has led to the questioning of the effectiveness of some practices (Woolf *et al.*, 1999) and has highlighted the need to question the way in which clinical decisions are made. The professional literature concerning evidence-based practice has been dominated by medicine, but many of the principles and problems are applicable to nursing.

Clinical guidelines are one method of disseminating research evidence to practitioners and have been used increasingly over the past decade (*see* Chapter 2). The current government reforms place particular emphasis on the use of clinical guidelines and the National Institute for Clinical Excellence (NICE) is now producing and disseminating national guidelines (*see* Chapter 12). Clinical governance, a framework of accountability, has also been introduced, which encourages guideline implementation (Royal College of Nursing, 1998).

Implementation of research findings, therefore, seems to be a rational thing to do, but in the health care setting such implementation is by no means the norm (Harrison, 1994). This is because changing people's behaviour is complex. In the field of health promotion a great deal of time, effort and money has been expended in trying to get people to change their behaviour in order to enhance their health, for example, encouraging people at risk of heart disease to eat a healthy diet or give up smoking. It seems there is little difference between this and the attempts to persuade practitioners to change their behaviour to improve their clinical practice. In each case there is an attempt to change what has become normal behaviour for that person and it is necessary to consider that change in the context within which it is to occur (*see* Chapter 4).

Effectiveness is a key component of quality that has been emphasized by UK health policy (NHS Executive, 1996; Department of Health, 1998; Wanless, 2002). Clinical effectiveness must be underpinned by research evidence. However, the use of evidence in clinical practice is not straightforward. There is difficulty in providing accessible, relevant and up-to-date scientific information to practising clinicians and there is recognition that in some clinical areas, such as nursing, the evidence is lacking. In 1995 Rosenburg and Donald highlighted:

1. the deterioration over time following qualification in doctors' knowledge and the associated failure of medical education to prevent this decline;
2. that the development of critical appraisal training is effective in keeping clinicians up to date;
3. that there have been developments in methods (notably meta-analysis), which make research more powerful and clinically relevant (*see* Chapter 2).

Evidence-based health care seeks to equip practitioners with the motivation and skills to use research evidence about the clinical effectiveness of diagnostic, treatment and management options in decisions about individual patients (Guyatt and Rennie, 1993). It also seeks to identify opportunities and barriers to the more widespread implementation of research findings into practice, as it is likely that variation represents considerable opportunity costs for the NHS (Grimshaw and Hutchinson, 1995). This concept acknowledges that in allocating resources to a particular service a sacrifice is made, in that an opportunity to obtain some other benefit is lost (Mooney *et al.*,1986) (*see* Chapter 5).

The use of research findings and evidence-based guidelines in primary care differs considerably from their use in secondary care. The lack of evidence on which to base primary care guidelines is often a barrier to describing a clearly defined management path (NHS Executive, 1997). Many primary care practitioners have large caseloads; this, coupled with increased patient expectations, often leads to a reactive rather then proactive approach to care, which might be more likely to incorporate new evidence into practice.

THE USE OF GUIDELINES TO CHANGE CLINICAL PRACTICE

Practice guidelines have been defined as: 'systematically developed statements to assist practitioner and patient decisions about appropriate health care for specific clinical circumstances' (University of Leeds, 1994:1). In the past, various strategies have been used to encourage practitioners to use the results of research to inform their practice, and many of these use evidence-based clinical guidelines as the starting point (Oxman, 1994). In 1994 Grimshaw and Russell systematically reviewed evaluations of clinical guidelines and concluded that. 'guidelines improve clinical practice and achieve health gains when introduced in the context of rigorous evaluations' (Grimshaw and Russell, 1994:). This work was extended and published as an *Effective Health Care* bulletin (University of Leeds, 1994). This bulletin examines whether guidelines can change the behaviour of health professionals and if so, how best to introduce them into clinical practice. It concludes that guidelines can change clinical practice and affect patient outcome, but the methods of development and implementation are important. If the guidelines took local circumstances into account, were disseminated by an active educational intervention, and implemented by specific patient reminders, they were more likely to change behaviour (see Box 6.1).

Since 1994 there has been considerable work on the process of development and utilization of guidelines (Feder *et al.*, 1999). The use of evidence to inform practice and using evidence-based guidelines for disseminating the research evidence seems eminently sensible. However, there are limitations to this approach that need to be recognized (Mead, 2000). In practice, the implementation of guidelines is not simple. Health care professionals are influenced by different forms of clinical knowledge and do not necessarily prioritize the 'evidence' obtained from randomized controlled trials. They may place more emphasis on experience and the social context within which they see the patient. Therefore, when considering the process of implementation of research evidence, it is important to explore how people are influenced

---

Box 6.1 Summary of *Effective Health Care* Bulletin: 'Implementing Clinical Guidelines' 1994

- Practice guidelines are systematically developed statements to assist practitioner and patient decisions about appropriate health care for specific clinical circumstances.
- The introduction of guidelines can change clinical practice and affect patient outcome. The way in which guidelines are developed, implemented and monitored influences the likelihood of adherence.
- Guidelines are likely to be more effective if they take into account local circumstances, are disseminated by an active educational intervention, and implemented by patient specific reminders relating directly to professional activity.
- Guidelines should be firmly based on reliable evidence of clinical and cost effectiveness. Recommendations should be explicitly linked to the evidence. Few national or local guidelines are sufficiently based on the evidence.
- National initiatives are needed to help to provide the evidence-base, which can be incorporated into national and local guidelines.
- Priority should be given to the development and introduction of local guidelines where nationally produced rigorous guidelines exist or where the evidence is readily available. Priority should be given to areas where current practice diverges from best practice providing significant gains in health.
- A coherent programme of research is needed to ensure that guidelines are used to their full potential.

(University of Leeds, 1994)

---

locally, because practice is made locally by different stakeholders with different interests, models of practice and views of the clinical knowledge base (Ferlie *et al.*, 1999). In summary then, it is of paramount importance that the care offered to patients is contextualized. As discussed in Chapters 3 and 4, a number of factors, including past experience, education and reading, the influence of colleagues' beliefs, and patients' own priorities and wishes, influence practitioners' decisions.

The remainder of this chapter describes specific examples of guideline implementation using data collected as part of a large multicentre research study. It explores how different primary health care teams used evidence-based guidelines for leg ulcer care within the former NHS Northern and Yorkshire Region and highlights some of the important issues for these community nursing teams. Although these data were collected as part of a research study, while a specific change strategy was being used, the issues are relevant and applicable to any practitioner working in community nursing.

THE NETWORK FOR EVIDENCE-BASED PRACTICE IN NORTHERN AND YORKSHIRE (NEBPINY) PROJECT

The aim of the NEBPINY project was to evaluate the effect of a multifaceted, evidence-based programme on the management of chronic diseases and patient outcomes. Three collaborating universities within the region recruited 53 general practices. Each practice chose to implement one of three evidence-based clinical guidelines, on either the management of persistent wheeze in adults, stable angina or venous leg ulceration. In this chapter data from the practices choosing to implement the venous leg ulcer guidelines will be presented, as this emerged as a specific area of nursing expertise. Figure 6.1 provides an overview of the full NEBPINY study.

Two facilitator/researchers worked with specific practices throughout the project. One was based in the northern part of the region and one in Yorkshire. Each recruited, audited and facilitated the same practices throughout the project. Of the 26 practices choosing to implement the leg ulcer guideline, 13 were randomized as control practices and were offered the intervention at the end of the project. The other 13 were randomized to the intervention arm of the trial; the qualitative data used in this chapter were collected during facilitated meetings in these practices.

The project intervention was the introduction of multidisciplinary evidence-based health care in individual general practices. It was a guideline implementation strategy that included:

- training to improve critical appraisal skills;
- audit with visual comparative feedback;
- provision of three copies of the evidence-based guidelines. These were in draft form at the time of the research, but are now published (Royal College of Nursing Institute, 1998);
- facilitation to support the application of the guidelines.

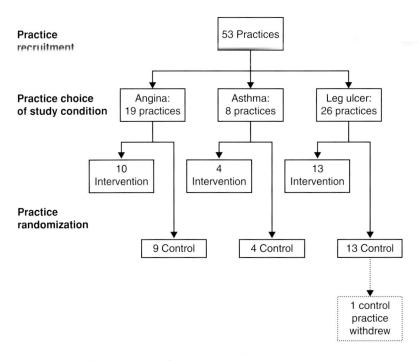

Fig. 6.1 *Overview of the NEBPINY project.*

Previous research has assessed the effectiveness of individual interventions to improve guideline implementation (Oxman, 1994; NHS Centre for Reviews and Dissemination, 1999). The NEBPINY project was seeking to use some of the interventions that had been shown to be most effective and, by combining them, to possibly enhance their effect. As discussed in Chapter 4, multifaceted approaches to practice development have been found to have most impact on change.

Clinical practice was audited at the beginning of the study and again after 6 months to measure compliance with the guidelines. These data were collected from the records of all patients with a venous leg ulcer, within the previous year, from each practice. The recording of three explicit recommendations (based on strong research evidence) from the guidelines was assessed in each record, both before and after the intervention. These were:

- assessment of the aetiology of a patient's leg ulcer using a Doppler machine;
- application of compression bandaging to a confirmed venous leg ulcer;
- advice to wear support stockings to prevent recurrence of healed ulcers.

These data were complemented by a qualitative study that collected data during group interviews conducted at facilitated meetings in the practices during the project. The aim of the qualitative analysis was to understand the process of guideline implementation and to assess the acceptability of the various elements of the intervention. These data also provided information about the context within which the guidelines were being implemented.

DETAILS OF THE NEBPINY INTERVENTION

Audit

The identification of patients with a venous leg ulcer in each practice proved problematic. Although most practices used computers, 'leg ulcer' was usually not coded in practice disease registers. Therefore, the practice nurses and community nurses were asked to recall, using diaries and nursing records, patients suffering from a venous leg ulcer. Once identified, a thorough search was made in the nursing documentation for a record of the three criteria. These were graphically presented to the practices, showing anonymous comparisons with other practices (Figs 6.2 and 6.3).

Critical appraisal training

Following collection of the audit data, two members of each practice were offered critical appraisal training. Although practices were encouraged to send participants from different professional groups, exactly who attended was their choice. This varied between practices: from many practices a general practitioner and a nurse (either district or practice nurse) attended. From others it was two nurses, usually a practice nurse and a district nurse. The workshop, which ran over one day, taught critical appraisal skills using the framework developed by the Critical Appraisal Skills

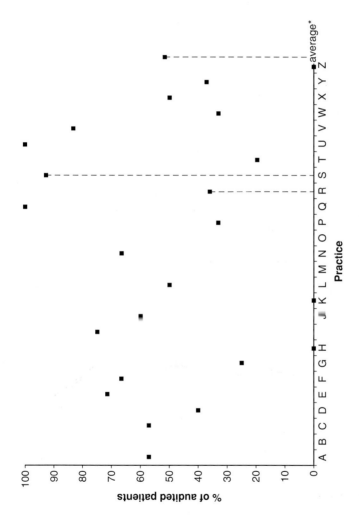

Fig. 6.2 *The percentage of patients for whom a Doppler test was found in the records before the intervention. *average, for all practices.*

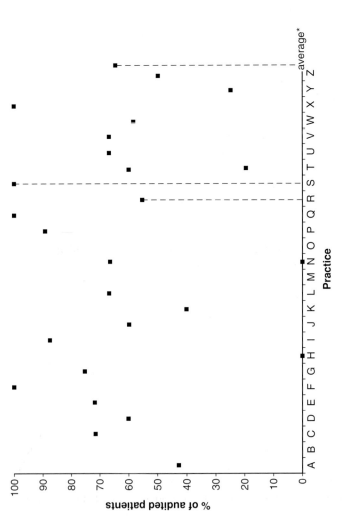

Fig. 6.3 *The percentage of patients for whom a record of compression bandaging was found before the intervention. *average, for all practices.*

Box 6.2 Critical Appraisal Skills Programme: 10 questions to help you make sense of a review

Are the results of the review valid?

1. Did the review address a clearly focused issue?
2. Did the authors look for the appropriate sort of papers?
3. Do you think the important relevant studies were included?
4. Did the review's authors do enough to assess the quality of the included studies?
5. If the results of the review have been combined, was it reasonable to do so?

What are the results?

6. What is the overall result of the review?
7. How precise are the results?

Will results help locally?

8. Can the results be applied to the local population?
9. Were all-important outcomes considered?
10. Are the benefits worth the harms and costs?

(CASP, 2002. Reproduced with permission. Current tools are available at:
http://www.phru.org.uk/~casp/resource/reviews.pdf)

Programme (CASP) in Oxford (Guyatt *et al.*, 1992) and introduced the clinical guidelines and their evidence base (*see* Chapter 12).

Specifically, the critical appraisal training taught the value of systematic reviews and the principles of meta-analysis (*see* Chapter 2). This was followed by the detailed appraisal of a systematic review of compression treatment for venous leg ulcers (Fletcher *et al.*, 1997), using the tool developed by CASP for appraisal of a systematic review, which had been adapted from a paper by Oxman (Oxman *et al.*, 1994) (*see* Box 6.2). This had been provided, with the programme, prior to the workshop.

The guidelines

The guidelines used for the management of venous leg ulceration were at the time in draft form and have since been published by the Royal College of Nursing (Royal College of Nursing Institute, 1998). McInnes *et al.* (2000) provide a description of the methods used to produce these guidelines. The guidelines made explicit the evidence-base for recommendations and the strength of that evidence (*see* Chapter 3) covering aspects of the assessment, management and dressing of venous leg ulcers. Table 6.1 gives details of some of the summary recommendations from the guidelines.

Facilitation

The facilitator/researchers involved in the fieldwork of the project both had backgrounds in nursing and experience of working in a primary care setting. They had a dual role of data collection for the project and facilitation of the implementation of

Table 6.1   *Some summary recommendations from the leg ulcer guidelines (Royal College of Nursing Institute, 1998:3)*

Recommendations	Strength of evidence*
All patients presenting with an ulcer should be screened for arterial disease by Doppler measurement of ABPI	I
Doppler measurement of ABPI should be done by staff who are trained to undertake this measure	II
Graduated multilayer high compression systems (including short stretch regimens), with adequate padding capable of sustaining compression for at least a week, should be the first line of treatment for uncomplicated venous leg ulcers (ABPI must be ≥ 0.8)	I
The compression system should be applied by a trained practitioner	II
Use of compression stocking reduces venous ulcer recurrence rates	I

* I, Strong evidence from at least one systematic review of multiple randomized controlled trials (RCTs); II, strong evidence from at least one properly designed RCT of appropriate size ABPI, ankle brachial pressure index.

the guidelines. Their role was to facilitate but not to direct the process of implementation. This involved supporting the work suggested by the practices and there was scope to carry out up to five visits per practice during the 6-month period, if requested. Other activities involved such things as information gathering on behalf of the practices, but providing specific training, for example, on the assessment of venous leg ulcers using Doppler examination, was outside this remit. Although offered, facilitation was not utilized to the full by many practices. The facilitation seemed to be important as a means of motivating practitioners to prioritize that particular area of work amongst the mountain of others competing for their time.

IMPLEMENTING EVIDENCE-BASED GUIDELINES FOR CARE OF PATIENTS WITH VENOUS LEG ULCER

The approach to practice development within the NEBPINY project was set by the research agenda, in that the intervention, as described above, was supplied to the practices. However, once recruited into the project, the practices were facilitated, not directed, which meant that the way they used the guidelines was organized by the team members. Consequently, the ways in which the guideline implementation was taken forward varied considerably between the practices. The following section describes the way in which two practices chose to implement the guidelines.

Case Study – Practice S

This practice, a large multi-site practice with a nurse manager involved in practice development, had a very committed community nursing team interested in leg ulcer management. I made contact initially with the practice through the nurse manager and visited first to carry out the audit. I collected the audit data mostly from the computer situated in the community office, although I also used patient care plans if information was missing from the computer record. This meant that during the time I was there I had opportunity to get to know the nurse manager and to meet most of the community nursing team. The nurse manager made a point of introducing me to the district nurses as they used the office.

I then met one of the district nurses as she attended the critical appraisal training with one of the general practitioners. The guidelines were given to participants at the workshop and by the time I visited the practice for the first meeting, the nurse, who had attended, had read them, and was sufficiently motivated to develop a summary of the guidelines for practice use. She discussed the summary with community nurse colleagues and this served to provide a degree of ownership of the process, which has been shown by previous studies to be important for guideline implementation (NHS Centre for Reviews and Dissemination, 1999). This summary document was then disseminated to all nurses and doctors within and attached to the practice. It was felt that this process was necessary to make the guidelines more accessible to all, making them simple to use and practical.

The nurse manager, the general practitioner and the district nurse who had attended the critical appraisal training, and several other district nurses and a student nurse attended the first meeting I held in the practice. There were no practice nurses at this meeting. These meetings were conducted using a semi-structured format to collect information from participants about the various aspects of the intervention, as well as being part of the implementation process. It also served to remind people of the training day and to disseminate the information to colleagues who had not attended. It also encouraged sharing of the content of the guidelines and any other information that others were aware of, for example, the existence of a patient information leaflet that had been developed by one of the nurses in the tissue viability clinic. As the facilitator I was non-directive, merely asking the group how they wished to take forward the implementation of the guidelines.

The group decided to run a workshop within the practice one lunchtime. The idea was to increase awareness and to encourage the nurses with little training in this area to identify their own training needs. The workshop was carried out using role-play, and emphasized the importance of holistic assessment of patients with a venous leg ulcer and the process of assessment of the venous leg ulcer using a Doppler machine. A further workshop was planned to cover bandaging techniques. Prior to this, the practice nurses in this practice had little experience of assessment of venous leg ulcers using a Doppler. During the workshop links between the practice nurses and the community nurses were improved. This resulted in the practice nurses feeling more able to contact the community nurses for advice or to carry out a Doppler examination for them. At a subsequent meeting the nurse manager said: 'I think we have managed to involve the practice nurses more in terms of actually requesting help from the district nurses, and actually getting involved in doing assessments.'

The nurse manager had already realized that there were training needs for this aspect of care but had not wanted to be directive, she wanted the nurses to identify their own needs. She took a very small role in the workshop, merely introducing the nurses carrying out the role-play and myself as researcher/facilitator.

The baseline audit results were already good for this practice prior to the intervention. There were a total of 14 patients who consented to take part in the research, of whom 93 per cent had a record of having been assessed using a Doppler machine and 100 per cent were currently treated with four-layer compression bandaging (*see* Figs 6.2 and 6.3). Of the five patients whose ulcers had healed, four had a record of having been advised to wear support stockings (80 per cent).

When compared to the results in other practices, the results for this practice were amongst the highest for the first two criteria. Giving advice to patients to wear support stockings to prevent recurrence following healing was less well done (*see* Chapter 3) and this was quickly identified by the district nursing team as a priority area for improvement and was addressed during the project; district nurse: 'we have been going back to check these patients after a month and then 6 months, I have got a note in my diary now to follow it up'.

There were several aspects in which this practice differed from many of the others participating in the study. It was the largest practice involved in the NEBPINY study, which meant that there were always patients receiving treatment for venous leg ulcers. Consequently, once the nurses were trained in venous leg ulcer management they were able to maintain their skills. In some of the smaller practices the nurses were concerned about maintaining their skills, as there were often no patients currently being treated for venous leg ulcers.

The community nurses in Practice S were all very committed, interested in venous leg ulcer care and were keen to improve healing times. Some of the nurses had gained their expertise initially by shadowing the specialist nurse at the dermatology clinic. This served not only to improve the skill base but also to improve links with the clinic for communication purposes. One example of the benefit of improved communication was the early awareness of some newly developed patient information leaflets.

The nurses in Practice S had easy access to the bandages needed for compression therapy. In many of the practices, at the time of the study, this was not the case. The four-layer bandages required for compression therapy were not then available on prescription. This meant that although many of the nurses knew this was the recommended method for healing venous leg ulcers they would try other dressings initially due to the cost of the bandages to the practice.

The nurses in Practice S had access to only one Doppler machine between them but, in spite of the fact that it was a multi-site practice, they shared it successfully between them and did not let this interfere with giving good care to patients. In some other practices the difficulty in obtaining a Doppler machine was cited as a reason for not being able to assess patients adequately. In some practices patients were referred to secondary care for assessment, the Doppler examination was carried out there and bandages supplied by the hospital; as one district nurse (Practice P) commented: 'we can get more supplies for them [patients] but not for anybody who is not under a dermatologist at the hospital'. This had the advantage of a clear diagnosis by skilled experts, but the disadvantages of lack of continuity of care for patients, and nurses' skills in Doppler examination were not well maintained.

The records were re-audited after 6 months to assess whether there had been any improvement in guideline compliance. The records of all patients reviewed in the first audit, who had consented to take part in the research, were scrutinized. The records for Practice S showed that 100 per cent of patients with venous leg ulcers had

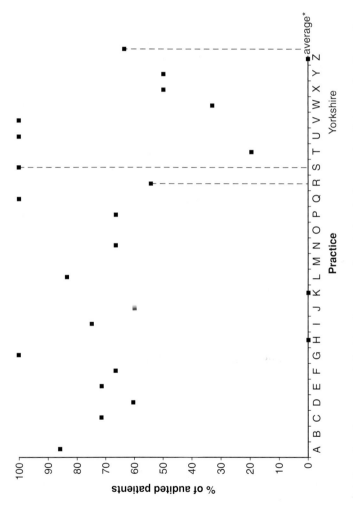

Fig. 6.4 *The percentage of patients for whom a record of a Doppler test was found after the intervention. *average, for all practices.*

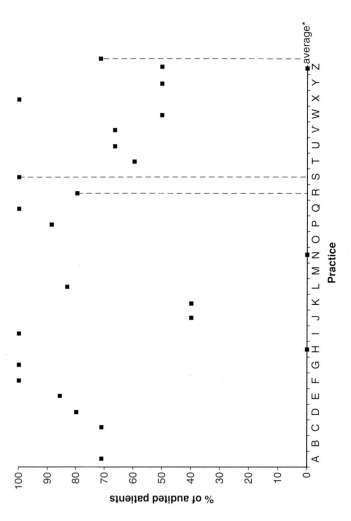

Fig. 6.5 *The percentage of patients for whom a record of compression bandaging was found after the intervention. *average, for all practices.*

been assessed by Doppler examination and 100 per cent were treated with compression bandaging (Figs 6.4 and 6.5). This was an improvement in the number of patients with a recording of a Doppler examination. Although the nurses had identified the use of compression stockings as an issue requiring their attention, the audit of existing patients did not show any change. It must, however, be appreciated that this represents just one patient who was still not receiving the care recommended by the guidelines or at least had no record of having been offered compression stockings. Audit of patients with newly healed ulcers within the intervention period showed that 100 per cent had been offered support stockings.

Principles extrapolated from case study of Practice S

To summarize, there are a number of principles demonstrated by this case study that may be of use to community practitioners attempting to implement change in practice using evidence-based guidelines:

- Audit with visual peer comparison (in the form of the graphs) and feedback, enabled easy identification of areas where improvement was needed. This provided positive reinforcement for nurses on areas that were being done well and, importantly, identified areas where improvement was needed.
- The nurses providing care were in control of, and able to change, their practice to improve quality of care. The process was not imposed or driven but facilitation enabled them to use imagination and innovation to address the areas identified by them as important.
- Sharing information and skills within the team raised standards of care. This would not have been possible without pre-existing good teamwork, communication and peer support.
- The district nursing team had liaised with practitioners in the clinic in secondary care to develop their skills initially. This informal use of resources within the area can often be quickly and easily arranged and has the additional benefit of improved links with secondary care and improved understanding of what happens to patients who are referred.
- By identifying their own needs and areas for improvement, the nurses were motivated to achieve improved care throughout the practice.

Case Study – Practice R

Practice R was a small rural practice in which the situation was very different. In this practice the nurses had responsibility for treating patients with venous leg ulcers and liaised with the general practitioners when a problem was identified. There was one practice nurse with expertise in assessing patients with leg ulcers. The other nurses, both district nurses and other practice nurses, referred patients with leg ulcers to her for assessment and changes in treatment, if possible, or continued providing the same treatment if this was not possible.

Compression bandaging had been initiated for patients with venous leg ulcers 2 years previously in this practice, stimulated by a request from a patient for the treatment! The lead practice nurse, who was experienced in assessment of leg ulcers, had recently come into post and had persuaded the general practitioners to buy a Doppler machine as she insisted that she could not apply compression bandaging without first carrying out a Doppler examination.

The nurses in this practice felt restricted in the number of bandages they could use. Although the general practitioners were willing to buy the four-layer bandaging system, there was a perception amongst the nurses that this was only acceptable as long as they did not use too many: '. . . you have got to decide really because the Profore, because we are having to buy them, it's costing the GP £100–£150 for every patient we put on them, so there is a limitation there as to how many they are going to allow us to do' (practice nurse). It is possible that this was only the nurses' perception and not what the GPs would have said had they been asked, because she went on to say: 'When we initially discussed it they [the GPs] were quite happy, but if all 21 patients were all on Profore then they wouldn't be very happy'.

In this practice very few patients with venous leg ulcers were referred to secondary care. This was due to the distance from the hospital and the reluctance of elderly patients to travel.

The practice was recruited to the research study through one of the general practitioners; my initial contact was the practice manager who organized the identification of patients with leg ulcers within the practice. I first met the practice nurse with expertise in leg ulcer care while carrying out the baseline audit. This enabled me to get to know her and to arrange the first facilitated meeting.

In this practice, the bulk of the care of patients with leg ulcers was recorded in the practice notes and was carried out by the practice nurse; care was occasionally carried out by the district nurses and then recorded in the district nursing notes. However, computers were used for prescribing and disease registers. These were used to identify patients with leg ulcers, with the help of the practice manager. The baseline audit results in this practice were not so good. There were a total of 11 patients identified at baseline (who consented to take part in the research); of these 36 per cent had a record of a Doppler examination and 55 per cent were treated with four-layer bandaging (see Figs 6.2 and 6.3). Four patients were identified who had ulcers that had healed and one of these had no record of being offered support stockings (75 per cent).

There were only three practice nurses present at the first facilitated meeting; both the general practitioner, who had attended the critical appraisal workshop, and the district nurses had been invited but were unable to attend. The meeting was carried out in the same format, as described previously, using a semi-structured interview schedule. The main problems identified during the first meeting were patient compliance with the four-layer bandaging system, co-morbidity, the lack of priority placed on the healing of leg ulcers and the financial constraints on the supply of bandages.

The nurses identified the need for a training session but this was never arranged. The problems were actually getting someone to do the training for so few people, and then maintaining the skills when only small numbers of patients were treated at any one time. I suggested arranging to visit the dermatology clinic at the local hospital for some training but this was not viewed positively. I sent a training video, purchased by the research project, but this was not used by many in the practice. When asked, the nurses chose not to have any further facilitation visits until the final audit. They did, however, identify the need to go through the notes for themselves. I made telephone contact twice with the lead practice nurse to supply the training video and to give them the details of the patient education leaflet in an effort to maintain enthusiasm for the work.

The second and final practice visit was well attended by both practice nurses and district nurses, but their perception was that little had been changed as a result of the project intervention: 'I think things had changed before we joined NEBPINY ... but I think it has helped to confirm what we are doing' (practice nurse).

However, the audit results showed improved use of Doppler assessment (55 per cent) and improved use of compression therapy (82 per cent). Of the four patients who had previously had healed ulcers, one still did not have a record of being offered stockings and of the two patients with newly healed ulcers one had a record of being offered stockings and the other did not (*see* Figs 6.4 and 6.5).

This practice demonstrated a lack of perception of the need to improve care, and there was little evidence of teamwork. One practice nurse was responsible for assessment and decision-making within the practice and there was nobody else with expertise to question her decisions. She took a conservative approach to the application of four-layer bandaging, which was compounded by the financial implications of their use, and her experience of poor patient compliance. This meant that the bandages were not applied consistently or optimally. The guidelines served to confirm to her that she was doing the right things and the low initial audit results appeared to have little impact as these were attributed by the nurses to poor recording: 'we felt there was a lot of discrepancy and we did think it was the actual reporting in the notes, because on the whole it seemed very low' (practice nurse).

When asked what she thought the project had achieved the lead practice nurse said: '... I would probably say that all we are doing is the right thing because we had moved forward quite a bit before we joined NEBPINY ... we had support stockings and compression bandages ... but it is right for some but not for everybody'.

When asked what they thought about the baseline audit results, one practice nurse said: 'on the whole we got the general feeling we were doing okay'.

My perception was that the patients treated using the guideline criteria were treated very well, but often support stockings were used instead of four-layer bandaging systems, due to the cost and poor compliance of patients. The evidence in the guidelines states that: 'There is reliable evidence that high compression achieves better healing rates than low compression.' But also that: 'the compression system should be applied by a trained practitioner' (Royal College of Nursing Institute, 1998). It may have been that using support stockings when untrained nurses were applying them (when the expert was not available) was deemed the safer option. On the other hand, it may be that the untrained nurses were unaware of the evidence that high compression is more effective than low compression.

The need for training, identified by the team, was not prioritized and, therefore, did not happen. It may have been due to lack of resources and the perception that it was unnecessary, as the one trained nurse could assess and plan the treatment for all the patients. The reluctance to apply four-layer bandages to some patients' venous leg ulcers may have been due to a lack of confidence in their skills and concern about an adverse event, or it could be that there was a lack of motivation to change traditional practice. Practitioners working in primary care, although part of a team, largely work alone, which may compound this problem: 'I think being a practice nurse you get very insular . . . you don't know whether you are doing the right thing or the wrong thing'. Yet, with the introduction of the post-registration education and practice (PREP) requirements in 1995 (UKCC, 2001) every nurse has a responsibility to keep up to date, regardless of the context in which they work.

This practice nurse did not use four-layer bandaging for patients with poor mobility: '. . . If the patient has got poor mobility I would never think of putting a Profore on, maybe more experienced staff would use it, but I personally would not . . .', yet these are the patients who would benefit most. It would seem this nurse was using intuition not evidence and was possibly concerned about litigation should a problem occur.

Principles extrapolated from the case study of Practice R

- The power and control of the nurse with some expertise in this practice may have deterred others in the practice from becoming trained in all aspects of leg ulcer care. This power was not necessarily sought by that particular nurse but conferred by others.
- This nurse came to the practice over 2½ years ago and had not had any further training in that time to update her skills, yet she was advising others. It is the responsibility of the nurses untrained in Doppler assessment and compression bandaging to identify their own training needs in order to develop competencies in these skills.
- The lack of a team approach to leg ulcer management is ultimately detrimental to patient care. If more people had been trained in the treatment of venous leg ulcers, then there would have been the opportunity for peer support if uncertainty arose about the treatment for a particular patient.

Summary of case studies

These two case studies have been presented to illustrate how differently teams within the practices, taking part in the NEBPINY project, were working prior to the research study. The teams responded in various ways to the research intervention package: the provision of critical appraisal training; evidence-based guidelines for the care of venous leg ulcers; audit and facilitation. It is interesting to note how these two practices varied in their use of the available resources. Other practices responded in different ways, but it is impossible to present all the practices as case studies. Some of the issues that emerged as themes from the qualitative analysis of all the practices choosing to implement the guidelines for venous leg ulcer are now considered.

QUALITATIVE DATA ANALYSIS

Qualitative data were collected from group interviews carried out at practice meetings. The meetings were all conducted using a semi-structured interview schedule, developed using the results of the feasibility study (Jones *et al.*, 1996). The participants were mostly district nurses and practice nurses, although general practitioners and other members of the primary health care team were present in some practices.

All meetings were recorded on to audiotape and were subsequently transcribed. Familiarization was achieved by repeatedly listening to tapes and reading transcripts enabling the main themes to be identified. The results of this analysis as they relate to the NEBPINY intervention are published elsewhere (Marshall *et al.*, 2001). There are, however, other themes that emerged from the study that are important to the process of change within a primary care setting and thus of interest to nurses delivering care to patients with venous leg ulcers. Some are illustrated by the case studies already reported, others are less explicit.

Patient-related factors

Nurses often described problems with compliance when attempting to deliver evidence-based care to patients with venous leg ulcers; in some cases this led to less optimal solutions, that were nevertheless acceptable to patients. One district nurse said: '. . . the type of patients we see are patients that are immobile, they are elderly and less likely to comply . . . we know what is the best form of treatment for them, but nine out of ten probably won't comply with what we suggest so we have to adapt'.

Nurses in many different practices identified reasons for non-compliance, including co-morbidity; the bandages being too hot or unsightly; inability to wear shoes comfortably; and difficulty in applying support stockings once the ulcer had healed. One practice nurse thought that if patients were better educated about why compression therapy was necessary, their compliance would be improved. Another thought that compliance was improved in the clinic situation as the patients heard evidence of healing from other patients. However, the patients attending clinics may well be different from those who are housebound, in that they are likely to be more mobile and possibly younger.

Several issues emerge from this analysis. First, the idea of professional power. There is the professional power of the nurse over the patient, which is illustrated by several nurses expecting patients to comply with their instructions without necessarily considering the patient's situation adequately. A practice nurse and a general practitioner recognized the importance of social contact for some patients: '. . . they have had them (leg ulcers) so long that they quite enjoy coming in and finding out what is going on here, it's a social contact, and they have had them so long they have accepted it really'. Some of the nurses described non-compliance as 'demoralizing' and found it frustrating to know the best treatment for venous leg ulcers but to be unable to achieve healing.

This raises two points: first, the evidence incorporated into guidelines is obtained from controlled situations and will not necessarily take into account such things as patient choice and quality of life or social aspects of care. Second, knowledge to inform practice is obtained from more than just the research evidence: the experience of previous similar situations, the influence of training and peers and knowledge of the patients' circumstances all contribute to the decision-making process (*see* Chapter 3).

Professional responsibility and resource constraints

In all the practices participating in the NEBPINY study, nurses were responsible for leg ulcer care. General practitioners were only involved if a problem such as infection was identified or a referral to secondary care was necessary. This, however, often meant that practice nurses were not supplied with the equipment with which to carry out optimum care. Access to a Doppler machine and getting supplies of four-layer bandages were often problematic for both practice nurses and district nurses. In some areas, the district nurses had access to these resources as they were provided by the community trust but the practice nurses could not access them. In some practices, the general practitioners bought the necessary equipment but there was a perceived need, often expressed by the nurses, to use them with caution, due to the cost. This illustrates a short-term view of expenditure of resources, as in the longer term savings could have been made by quicker healing times and the use of fewer bandages and less nursing time.

Many nurses were trained in assessment of patients with leg ulcers, Doppler examination and application of four-layer bandaging, but many were not. In the case study Practice S, there had been informal training arranged, but in other areas, the trusts had provided training. In practices where there was good communication and teamwork, once a number of nurses were trained, skills were shared to give better quality care. It is the responsibility of the individual nurse to ensure she is competent to carry out tasks expected within her role (UKCC, 1992; Nursing and Midwifery Council, 2002) but also the responsibility of the employer (Royal College of Nursing, 1998).

CONCLUSION

The use of the NEBPINY guidelines

The use of the guidelines within the practices varied immensely. Several practices were already using local guidelines issued to them by their health authority or the community trust. These practices did not achieve much change in practice, as the guidelines already in use were very similar to the national guidelines (Royal College of Nursing Institute, 1998) and the process of change had already occurred. In most practices where the guidelines had been used, a summary had been produced for practice use.

The guidelines were perceived by the nurses to provide a framework to supplement their clinical judgement and were believed to ensure consistency and promote a team approach to care. Many practitioners expressed the view that guidelines should be used flexibly and should be adapted for particular patients: 'the guidelines are there as guidelines but obviously you have got to address them in different ways to different people, but it's nice to have something there to work from'.

The use of audit

The use of audit with comparative visual feedback of results served to promote change in some practices with poor results. In others, particularly if the results were perceived to be a result of poor recording, it had little influence on practice. In practices where results were high, some were motivated to improve still further whereas some practitioners expressed complacency and did not improve.

Facilitation

It is very difficult to assess whether the facilitation process was useful or not. Primary care teams were asked the question by the facilitators and this felt very uncomfortable. This may have elicited more positive replies than if asked by someone externally (as discussed in Chapter 5, common courtesy can sometimes get in the way of objective evaluation). Also, as the approach used was very non-directive, with the aim of encouraging the teams to take the initiative themselves and empowering them to make the changes, the facilitation should not have been intrusive and was, therefore, possibly more difficult for participants to evaluate. There were few spontaneous references to the facilitation process. However, when asked, the responses were positive, and for most practices it did prompt them to implement actions they had identified in previous meetings when they knew another visit was due. One nurse said: 'I think you are more likely to follow guidelines and be involved when you actually meet someone face-to-face to discuss it'.

There are many strategies for change that have the potential to facilitate the implementation of evidence-based guidelines in primary health care. It is clear that, due to the complexity and variety of situations, there will never be one 'magic bullet' that will be successful in every case. The existing context needs to be taken into account and an initial assessment of the potential barriers to implementation made in order to identify ways in which they might be overcome at the beginning of the process. I hope that by presenting these case studies and some qualitative findings of the broader research study I may have given practitioners inspiration and ideas that may be used in a variety of situations in their own practice. There are a number of factors that seem to be important, and have been highlighted by this research process, that may be useful to community practitioners seeking to implement guidelines in their own practice:

Key points for practice development initiatives

Principles extrapolated from the NEBPINY study

- There is a need to take professional responsibility and to be accountable for nursing decisions regarding patient care. This must combine clinical expertise and the best available evidence, while taking account of the patient's priorities. In many cases, the practitioner's role will be to present information on available options to the patient, enabling them to make an informed choice.
- All community practitioners should ensure that they have undertaken training and have the skills and competencies needed to deliver high-quality care. When caring for patients with venous leg ulcers these include Doppler assessment and bandaging techniques.

- In order to achieve maximum quality improvement, the process of guideline implementation, which is complex, should be owned by the practitioners delivering the care to the patients.
- The use of audit with comparative feedback can motivate some practice teams. This may be carried out anonymously within Primary Care Trusts but must include a commitment to complete the full quality-improvement cycle.
- Facilitation is particularly useful to encourage a team to concentrate on one area of care as a priority and can encourage the team to meet deadlines set by themselves. It is useful to provide summary notes of meetings for circulation to all present at the meeting and others concerned who were unable to attend.
- Non-directive facilitation may be most effective. The use of positive feedback to motivate practitioners further and opportunities for them to identify their own needs can be effective.
- The use of critical appraisal training can enhance nurses' appreciation of the way guidelines are produced and their evidence-base. The application of critical appraisal skills can save time and enable practitioners to identify which 'evidence' they should consider implementing in practice. Good course preparation is essential, and ensuring relevance to practice is likely to motivate and thus enhance use of the skills. Managers and practitioners should consider skills such as these as important as clinical skills.
- For maximum quality improvement, change in practice must occur within the whole team. It is essential to ensure that the main stakeholders and opinion leaders are involved.
- Any change will require resources, if only time for meetings. The relevant resources or potential sources should be identified and should be considered at the planning stage.
- Knowledge from research findings is perceived and prioritized in different ways by different people; this may produce a barrier to the implementation of evidence-based guidelines.
- Practitioners need to understand the dynamics of professional power, particularly within the professional–patient relationship. If power relations are not taken into account, both changing professional practice and patient behaviour will be difficult.
- Evidence-based guidelines are produced based on a specific population of patients. Therefore, sometimes the provision for individualized patient care does not fit comfortably with guideline recommendations. Clinical judgement must be used in conjunction with the evidence, also taking account of other aspects such as patient preferences and the value placed on various aspects of quality of life.
- Visible improvement of patient outcomes (e.g. healing of a leg ulcer) provides strong motivation to change practice. Therefore if the outcome in question is not so visible, use of epidemiological methods to measure and present outcomes may be considered. Within a Primary Care Trust this may be achieved by liaison with public health personnel.

ACKNOWLEDGEMENTS

I would like to thank Paula Mead (researcher/facilitator) for her valuable comments on this manuscript and Daphne Russell (statistician) for her analysis of the audit data and production of the graphs. The NEBPINY study was designed and developed by I. Russell, A. Hutchinson, B. McAvoy, A.P. Roberts, A. Wilson and K. Jones. K. Jones designed the qualitative component of the study, and analysis was carried out by E. Kaba, P. Mead and J. Marshall. The interpretations used in this chapter are those of the author.

REFERENCES

CASP 2002. Critical Appraisal Skills Programme Appraisal Tools, Milton Keynes Primary Care Trust (http//:www.phru.org.uk/~casp/index.htm).

Department of Health 1998 *A First Class Service*. The Stationery Office, London.

Feder G, Griffiths C, Eldridge S and Spence M 1999 Effect of postal prompts to patients and general practitioners on the quality of primary care after a coronary event (POST): randomised controlled trial. *British Medical Journal* 318(7197): 1522–6.

Ferlie E, Wood M and Fitzgerald L 1999 Some limits to evidence-based medicine: a case study from elective orthopaedics. *Quality in Health Care* 8: 99–107.

Fletcher A, Cullum N and Sheldon T 1997 A systematic review of compression treatment for venous leg ulcers. *British Medical Journal* 315: 576–80.

Grimshaw JM and Hutchinson A 1995 Clinical practice guidelines – do they enhance value for money in health care? *British Medical Bulletin* 51: 927–40.

Grimshaw JM and Russell IT 1994 Achieving health gain through clinical guidelines II: Ensuring guidelines change medical practice. *Quality in Health Care* 3: 45–52.

Guyatt GH and Rennie D 1993 Users' guides to the medical literature. *Journal of the American Medical Association* 270: 2096–7.

Guyatt G, Cairns J, Churchill D, Cook D, Haynes B, Irvine J, Levine M, Nishikawa I, Sachett D, Brill Edwards P, Gerstein H, Gibson J, Jaeschke R, Kerigan A, Neville A and Panju A 1992 Evidence-Based Medicine Working Group. Evidence-based medicine: A new approach to teaching the practice of medicine. *Journal of the American Medical Association* 268(17): 2420–5.

Harrison S 1994 Knowledge into practice: what's the problem? *Journal of Management in Medicine* 8(2): 9–16.

Jones K, Wilson A, Russell I, Roberts A, O'Keefe C, McAvoy B, Hutchinson A, Dowell A and Benech I 1996 Evidence-based practice in primary care. *British Journal of Community Nursing* 1: 276–80.

Marshall J L, Mead P, Jones K, Kaba E and Roberts AP 2001 The implementation of venous leg ulcer guidelines: process analysis of the intervention used in a multi-centre, pragmatic, randomized, controlled trial. *Journal of Clinical Nursing* 10(6): 758–66.

McInnes E, Cullum N, Nelson AE, Luker K and Duff LA 2000 The development of a national guideline on the management of leg ulcers. *Journal of Clinical Nursing* 9: 208–17.

Mead P 2000 Clinical guidelines: promoting clinical effectiveness or a professional minefield? *Journal of Advanced Nursing* 31(1): 110–16.

Mooney GH, Russell EM and Weir RD 1986 *Choices for Health Care: A Practical Introduction to the Economics of Health Provision*. Studies in Social Policy. Macmillan, London.

NHS Centre for Reviews and Dissemination 1999 Getting evidence into practice. *Effective Health Care* bulletin. NHS Centre for Reviews and Dissemination, University of York, York.

NHS Executive 1996 *Promoting clinical effectiveness: A framework for action in and through the NHS*. NHSE, Leeds.

NHS Executive 1997 *R&D in Primary Care. National Working Group Report*. (Chair Professor D. Mant). Department of Health, London.

Nursing and Midwifery Council 2002 *Code of professional conduct*. Nursing and Midwifery Council, London.

Oxman A 1994 *No Magic Bullets: A Systematic Review of 102 Trial Interventions to Help Healthcare Professionals Deliver Services More Effectively or Efficiently*. North East Thames Health Authority, London.

Oxman AD, Cook DJ and Guyatt GH 1994 Users guides to the medical literature. VI. How to use an overview. *Journal of the American Medical Association* 272: 1367–71.

Rosenburg W, Donald A 1995 Evidence Based Medicine: An Approach to Clinical Problem-Solving *BMJ* 310: 1122–26.

Royal College of Nursing 1998 *Guidance for Nurses on Clinical Governance*. Royal College of Nursing, London.

Royal College of Nursing Institute 1998 *Clinical Practice Guidelines for the Management of Patients with Venous Leg Ulcers: Recommendations for Assessment, Compression Therapy, Cleansing, Debridement, Dressings, Contact Sensitivity*. Royal College of Nursing and Centre for Evidence-Based Nursing, School of Nursing Midwifery and Health Visiting, University of Manchester. RCN Publishing, London.

Sackett DL, Rosenberg WMC, Gray JAM, Haynes RB and Richardson WS 1996 Evidence based medicine: what it is and what it isn't. *British Medical Journal* 312: 71–2.

UKCC (United Kingdom Central Council for Nursing, Midwifery and Health Visiting) 1992 *Scope of Professional Practice*. UKCC, London.

UKCC (United Kingdom Central Council for Nursing, Midwifery and Health Visiting) 2001 *The PREP Handbook*. UKCC, London.

University of Leeds 1994. Implementing clinical practice guidelines: can guidelines be used to improve clinical practice. *Effective Health Care* bulletin. University of Leeds, Leeds.

Wanless D 2002 *Securing Our Future Health: Taking a Long-Term View*. Final Report. HM Treasury, London. http://www.hm-treasury.gov.uk/Con...anless/consult_wanless_final.cfm

Woolf SH, Grol R, Hutchinson A, Eccles M and Grimshaw J 1999 Potential benefits, limitations, and harms of clinical guidelines. *British Medical Journal* 318: 527–30.

7

Local guidelines: Development and implementation in minor injury units

Hilary Gledhill

Purpose of this chapter

- To describe the need for local guidelines.
- To describe the process of guideline development.
- To describe the processes used to support change.

INTRODUCTION

Guidelines have been found to have the potential to achieve significant change in practice (University of Leeds, 1994). The *Effective Health Care* bulletin published by the University of Leeds (1994) indicates that there is evidence that locally produced guidelines, or national guidelines that have been adapted to the local context, have more impact on practice. However, development of guidelines is only half the story: to be effective guidelines need to be incorporated into the day-to-day practice of individuals. In their summary of the evaluation of the North Thames Region programme of 17 projects aimed at introducing evidence-based guidelines, Wye and McClenahan (2000:26) conclude: 'Implementation is the real work: guidelines are not enough'. A comment from one of the projects sums up the danger that the focus of the project may become the production of a glossy document rather than making a change to patient care: 'With hindsight, we feel that we may have succumbed to the temptation to produce an impressive document at the expense of the main objective, changing practice' (Wye and McClenahan, 2000:27).

This chapter is, therefore, concerned with both these elements: the process of producing guidelines and the change process involved both to enable the guidelines to be produced and to support their use in practice; and takes you through a journey resulting in the implementation of evidence-based guidelines into the minor injury units (MIUs) attached to two community hospitals. During the period of this project I was the nurse manager in one of the community hospitals.

The chapter discusses the approach used to involve and motivate the team of practitioners and ensure that motivation was sustained throughout the development of the guidelines. The development and implementation of the guidelines is discussed, with some of the issues that arose from undertaking this project, which ultimately elongated the whole process.

The nurses' attitudes to change, the role of the nurse manager in the change process, and the power of a robust system of clinical supervision to support and guide clinicians through change are then explored. The chapter concludes by reflecting on the process used; the benefits to clinical practice; areas for future development; and, from my own perspective as the nurse manager overseeing the process, identifies parts of the change process which, on reflection, I may have approached differently.

PROJECT BACKGROUND

A number of local issues led to the establishment of this project, including:

- distance of the MIUs from the local accident and emergency department (A&E);
- wide range in severity of conditions, particularly in holiday periods;
- traditional practice based on 'treatment books';
- differences in practice between the two units.

The two MIUs involved in the project were located in small seaside towns on the east Yorkshire coast. Both were integrated into the local community hospital in each of the towns. They were not only housed within the same building, but the same nursing staff that worked on the adjacent in-patient community ward, also, at the 'ring of a bell', attended to the person presenting at the unit. The MIUs were chiefly nurse-led, with medical cover being provided by local general practitioners on request. Advice and support were also sought as necessary from the nearest A&E department.

Other members of the primary health care team were also based at both community hospitals, including district nurses, health visitors and community psychiatric nurses. They were also called on for their expert knowledge by staff in the MIU, providing support and advice when necessary. As Tucker (2001) describes, the important role of the community hospital as part of an integrated primary health care service is becoming increasingly important, reinforcing the need for such staff to be involved in practice development processes.

As both of the MIUs were situated in seaside towns, the number of people attending fluctuated. Holidaymakers and day-trippers would cause an increase in service users during the summer months. Many of these visitors attended with complex medical problems more suited to a medical assessment but still requiring some form of nursing assessment to be undertaken. Visitors to the area would not always understand the role of a MIU and would sometimes present with conditions that required attendance at the A&E department 18 miles away. As both of the hospitals were in rural areas, lack of availability of an ambulance to transport these patients often meant that the nursing staff would have to deal with problems that they were neither equipped nor trained for, while awaiting the arrival of an ambulance.

In this context, both MIUs had produced their own 'treatment books' covering a variety of topics, including dog bites, abdominal pain and overdose. The topics covered were few; they had a tendency to be task orientated and medical in origin. There was no supporting evidence to underpin the information and often no indication of how current the information was. There was no indication that the information was supporting 'best practice' and consequently the information was rarely referred to, resulting in the nursing staff providing a service based on their own experience, which resulted in variations in treatments and subsequently variations in outcomes. Such an approach was clearly not consistent with a cost-effective, evidence-based approach to practice (NHS Executive, 1996). Rarely could anyone justify why there were obvious variations in practice. The lack of consistency in practice raised ethical concerns amongst the nursing team about members of the public receiving a different service dependent upon whom they presented to rather than what they presented with. This ethical dilemma proved to be a key factor in getting the team on board with the proposed change.

MIUs can by nature be clinically challenging areas. Reasons for patients of all ages presenting at an MIU can range from a simple cut that requires cleansing to a mental health crisis, crushing chest pain or injuries resulting from abuse. Consequently, the nurses working within these units have to develop a complex set of skills. To facilitate the development of these skills there needs to be in place a framework providing support, clinical supervision, continuous professional development and training and education to enable the nurse to work confidently while developing and enhancing the skills required. In 1997, at the time of the project, no external education course was available for nurses working in MIUs and training was provided in-house from the community trust training department and in the community hospitals by the local GPs. As there was limited opportunity for nurses to enhance their clinical skills, it was considered that the production of a robust set of evidence-based clinical guidelines could be used to support nurses working in MIUs, and could begin to make inroads into standardizing the care offered in the MIUs.

PLANNING THE PROJECT

The decision having been made that clinical guidelines would assist in the provision of high-quality care, the process of guideline development commenced. Practice development in the community hospitals was led by the head of profession for registered nurses in the community trust. She chaired the professional development group, which consisted of lead clinicians from both of the community hospitals, who undertook work on this project when clinical demands on their time were less. This group worked in collaboration with the manager of the locality within which both community hospitals were situated. In order to ensure the guidelines were going to be used by the clinicians who worked in the MIUs, it was felt by the professional development group and the locality manager that staff should have ownership of the guidelines. This view mirrored the recommendations of the *Effective Health Care* bulletin (University of Leeds, 1994), although there is other evidence that suggests that in some practice areas, local ownership may not be as crucial as previously thought (Sivakumar and Haigh, 2000). Lead clinicians who worked in the MIUs volunteered to participate in the process and a project group was established. As Eve *et al.* (1997) comment, a working group or committee is often established, particularly where change is led from the top of an organization, to take forward change, as 'the committee' is a familiar and, therefore, comfortable setting for managers.

The process of developing and subsequently implementing the guidelines had to be planned and the process for the change agreed. All of the staff and senior managers needed to be aware of the change process that had been agreed, the perceived benefits to patient care and clinical outcomes, and be clear about their roles/responsibilities within the identified change.

To begin with, the group devised a project plan to ensure that the guidelines were developed in an expedient fashion. A framework was developed incorporating identified timescales indicating when completion of each guideline was expected (Sanderson and Gledhill, 1999). This part of the process was led by the head of profession for Registered General Nurses (RGNs) in the community trust who was the professional lead for the community hospitals and thus for the staff within the MIUs. She assisted the group in prioritizing the guidelines and finalizing the format in which they were to be presented. Once the topics and the format for presentation had been decided, it was then the task of the team to seek out supporting evidence and to devise the guideline. Once the guideline was in an acceptable format it was the task of the professional lead to seek advice from those considered experts in the area of each particular guideline, for example medical staff, the health promotion department or the mental health team, for their views on the guidelines. As Tingle (1997a) comments, such endorsement is important in the utilization of guidelines: 'To be viewed as proper in a legal context, clinical guidelines must reflect a responsible body of Medical or Nursing opinion, i.e. other doctors or nurses have created and used the guidelines in the same or similar way'.

Once the guidelines had been completed they were to be incorporated into a handbook for each of the MIUs.

What is a guideline?

Before any of the above work could commence it became obvious to the group that they would need to define the purpose of the guidelines to be included in the handbook (*see* Chapters 2 and 6 for a more extensive discussion of this subject). Following discussion and consideration of information on guidelines, including the *Effective Health Care* bulletin (University of Leeds, 1994) on guideline implementation, the definition given in Box 7.1 was agreed by the group.

Developing the guidelines

The remit of the group was to produce a handbook of guidelines that would:

Box 7.1 Guideline definition

The guidelines contained within this handbook for use in the Minor Injury Departments of the Community Hospitals are intended to:

- act as the appropriate decision-making pathway process;
- reflect the degree of expertise that the nurse is expected to have in terms of clinical and decision-making skills;
- guide the process of decision-making but be flexible enough to allow the experienced nurse to use judgement within the the UKCC (1992a) *Scope of Professional Practice*;
- facilitate autonomous decision-making.

- be evidence based;
- reflect the degree of expertise that the nurse working in the department was expected to have;
- guide the decision-making process but be flexible enough to allow the experienced nurse to use judgement within the UKCC (1992a) *Scope of Professional Practice*;
- reflect the level of service available in a hospital with no on-site doctors.

The next phase of the project was for the teams to identify the 20 guidelines that needed to be developed as a priority. Priority areas were identified from the numbers of patients presenting at the MIUs with a particular condition, areas of practice in which variance in treatments occurred the most, and areas where we knew there was already evidence that could underpin the practice (*see* Box 7.2 for examples of the topics). Once the topics had been identified, the group then began its task of finding the evidence that would underpin the guideline, but prior to this we had to decide what we meant by evidence and locate a tool to help us evaluate the different types of evidence.

Following team discussions, with regard to 'What is evidence?', it was identified by the group that in many areas of practice there was a lack of supporting evidence. Where there was evidence, it was often variable in quality, and sometimes the proposed practice was not practical in a primary care setting. These conclusions are

---

Box 7.2 Examples of the guideline topics

- Head injury
- Human bites
- Animal bites
- Burns
- Abdominal pain
- Chest pain
- Management of diabetes
- Overdose

supported by the conclusions of the Mant report (NHS Executive, 1997), which reviewed the state of primary care research. The report found that research evidence relevant to primary care was lacking in many areas, and recommended that greater investment in primary care research was necessary. Through these discussions the team came to the view that the supporting information to underpin the guidelines could consist of much more than the available research. As discussed in Chapter 3, there is a wide range of information available, including research, professional experience and patient or carer experiences, to name but a few.

Cullum (1998) suggests that guidelines must be based on quality systematic reviews where there is plenty of robust research. However, given the dearth of research evidence, it was decided that a more pragmatic approach had to be taken. With this in mind, the group began collecting the results of audits, projects, past practice and expert views, which, with the evidence from research, would be used to underpin the selected guidelines for inclusion in the handbook.

To enable us to evaluate the value of the material we had amassed, we identified that we needed a tool that would:

- allow us to recognize that although research is clearly some of the best type of evidence, it is not the only type;
- enable us to make statements about the quality of information used to underpin each guideline;
- allow us to identify where research is poor and influence the research agenda; and
- ensure a systematic approach to retrieving and analysing information.

We decided as a group to use the hierarchy of evidence produced by the NHS Centre for Reviews and Dissemination (1996) (*see* Chapter 3), which we modified slightly for our use (Box 7.3).

For each guideline topic, a thorough literature review was conducted. The search for literature was undertaken by the head of professions for RGNs, who undertook searches of databases, including the Cochrane database, Medline and Cinhal (Sanderson and Gledhill, 1999) (*see* Chapters 2 and 12 for access to these databases and web sites providing advice on the development of guidelines). Based on this information, together with the views of experts and any available audits, a draft guideline was drawn up. The project group then reviewed the guideline, made any amendments and, using the hierarchy of evidence, the quality of the information on

---

Box 7.3 Evidence-based guidelines and the hierarchy of evidence

⇒ Level 1: NHS Centre for Reviews and Dissemination or Cochrane database review
⇒ Level 2: Other reviews of the research
⇒ Level 3: Large-scale, well-designed primary studies, randomized-controlled trials and other controlled trials
⇒ Level 4: Large-scale primary studies using other methods
⇒ Level 5: The opinions and experience of respected authorities based on clinical experience, descriptive studies and reports

(Adapted from NHS Centre for Reviews and Dissemination, 1996)

which the guideline was based was rated. This rating was then displayed on the guideline with supporting references (*see* Note 1).

Applying the guidelines

Lead staff from the MIUs had been involved in developing the guidelines and staff had been kept informed of the progress of the project throughout the development phase. Once the guidelines had been agreed, the group decided that, to assist the implementation phase, each trained nurse working within the MIUs should be introduced to the guideline handbook on an individual basis. This introduction was undertaken by the unit managers. All staff were given the opportunity to discuss the contents and their responsibility with regard to their use. The guidelines covered a range of topics, from stings to asthma, and incorporated changes in practice, covering, in some instances, the directive to administer medication. It was important for the nurse not only to feel comfortable using them but to be confident with them. Utilization of the guidelines was facilitated by day-to-day discussions and support offered by myself and the project team.

CHANGE MECHANISMS

As suggested in the introduction, the development of guidelines involves considerable change in practice, and this process needs to be undertaken with sensitivity (*see* Chapter 4). In the present project the nurse manager was instrumental in the change process, and clinical supervision provided the support system within which the issues concerning the utility of the guidelines for practice could be discussed.

The role of the nurse manager

My role as the manager was to facilitate the change. I had to ensure that the staff identified to be a part of the project team were given time away from hands-on clinical duties to ensure that they had protected time to progress the project. Part of my role in this process was to assist the team in the decision-making process of identifying the priority guidelines and how they could be presented in a user-friendly format. I had to ensure peer support for those involved in the project. All of the staff in the community hospitals/MIUs were informed of the purpose and progress of the project. They were all involved in the debate regarding the need for practice to change, the benefits not only to the patients, but to the nursing staff themselves. They all understood the process being used and believed it would produce the results required. I had to ensure that while staff took time out to debate and research the issues raised, the motivation to ensure the agreed change took place and the ultimate aim of implementing evidence-based guidelines was not lost.

Clinical supervision

It became clear from the outset that some of the issues raised within the nursing team were very complex. These issues suggested that what at first had appeared to be a simple project with a relatively short timescale, was going to be anything but. Box 7.4 provides some examples of the complex organizational issues identified by the staff.

Some of the issues raised did not have easy solutions. They took so long to debate, often without a clear outcome, that they in themselves became a barrier to the change. These issues led to a feeling of demotivation with a potential to undermine what we were trying to achieve. It often felt as if the whole service was under threat. Small groups of nursing staff would form in huddles debating clinical issues, which the change was identifying as a potential risk. With no one to facilitate these informal groups, and subsequently seek action, other leaders began to emerge, some with a positive attitude to the change, others that were not so positive. The latter became identified as possible saboteurs to the success of the project. These informal debates between staff were in some ways useful, however, as they allowed staff to air their views in a non-threatening way, but they needed a forum for debate to allow all team members the opportunity to participate and jointly seek solutions to the arising problems. This forum was provided through clinical supervision (see Chapter 2). Clinical supervision sessions were the vehicle used to develop some of the issues that the project group identified, and were held regularly throughout the change.

Clinical supervision had only recently been introduced to the team. Following training in this area, I had undertaken a series of presentations to the team, defining what clinical supervision was, its purpose and the various models of delivering clinical supervision that were available. Through these presentations the group debated and agreed to adopt the definition of clinical supervision shown in Box 7.5.

The team discussed all of the perceived benefits of meeting in this way. It was important at this time to ensure that staff agreed ground rules for clinical supervision sessions, such as confidentiality, and that they recognized the differences

---

Box 7.4 Organizational and other issues raised by staff

- Accessibility of appropriate resources, including medical staff; nurses; equipment and support services.
- Legal aspects of nursing.
- Grading issues.
- Training issues.
- The role of the nurse practitioner.
- The level of service being provided in the MIUs.

Box 7.5 Definition of clinical supervision

A term used to describe a formal process of professional support and learning which enables individual practitioners to develop knowledge and competence, assume responsibility for their own practice and enhance consumer protection and safety of care in complex situations. It is central to the process of learning and to the expansion of the Scope of Professional Practice and should be seen as a means of encouraging self-assessment and analytical and reflective skills.

(Department of Health, 1993)

between clinical supervision and other meetings that they attended as a team; for example, team meetings where practical issues about the day-to-day running of the team were discussed, but no attempts were made to develop areas of practice.

We debated different issues and decided what we required from clinical supervision and which issues we wished to debate in this forum. Clinical supervision was described by Proctor (1986 cited by Kohner, 1994) as performing three interactive functions: formative, restorative and normative. The formative function describes the educative role of clinical supervision, and is about developing the practitioner's knowledge and skills. The restorative function describes the supportive help to practitioners that can be provided by supervision; and the normative function is the quality control component of supervision through which professional standards are scrutinized and maintained. In developing clinical guidelines it was clear that all three functions of clinical supervision would need to be met.

Once we had agreed the benefits of clinical supervision and the role and responsibility of the supervisor, we began to look at the different models available (Houston, 1990):

- one-to-one with a supervisor from your own discipline;
- one-to-one peer supervision (with people of a similar grade, expertise from within the team or external to the team);
- group supervision (multigrade consisting of the regular working team).

The group identified that all of the above models were already in place, in different areas, either through existing meetings or through an informal process that had grown from within the team, who had historically always been supportive of each other. A different approach was felt necessary to ensure that what was already in place would continue, but which would give some structure to the process, allowing all team members to be involved.

The framework to deliver clinical supervision in a community hospital setting began to evolve (Fig. 7.1).

It was felt that a mix of models would enable the continuation of the good practice that already existed, but also, by making clinical supervision a formal process and part of the organizational culture, would enable practice to develop within a supportive framework. It was also anticipated that having a mix of different models for clinical supervision in the community hospital would allow individuals to learn and develop in their practice in the setting that they found most helpful.

Following this period of debate, it was agreed that this framework to clinical supervision incorporating a number of different models would be adopted in the community hospitals. It was anticipated that clinical supervision would:

- enhance the practice of nurses;
- improve patient care;
- encourage professional growth;
- develop the confidence of nurses;
- broaden the thinking of individuals;
- improve team relationships.

The proposed clinical supervision framework needed to be tested. Staff were not convinced that it would offer the outcomes expected. Although we did not realize it

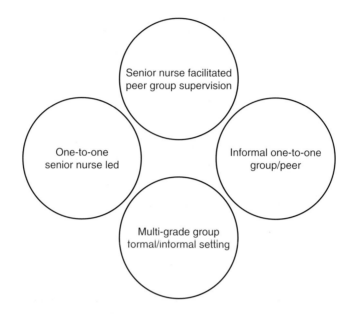

Fig. 7.1 *Framework for clinical supervision in a community hospital.*

at the outset of the guidelines project, the proposal to implement evidence-based guidelines proved to be the ultimate test for the clinical supervision. The clinical supervision meetings enabled staff to debate many issues concerned with the implementation of the guidelines and, thus, the clinical supervision process facilitated the development and introduction of the guidelines. Equally, the development of the guidelines reinforced the introduction of clinical supervision.

Questioning guideline development and implementation

In the clinical supervision sessions many issues relevant to the introduction of guidelines were discussed, including the following.

'We are hands-on nurses; we don't have the time to work on projects away from our patients'

Trying to identify time-out proved to be one of the main obstacles, particularly as we had chosen to start the project during the summer months when the workforce numbers were low due to an increase in annual leave. Taking clinical staff away from practice is always difficult: 'the patient always comes first' being the attitude adopted not only by some managers at the time but by the staff themselves. Lack of time spent on staff development away from direct patient care may be one factor restricting the development of nursing practice. I had many debates with the nursing and medical staff about the need to develop evidence-based nursing practice, thus to ensure that the standard of nursing would be of the same and, in some cases, of more value to the patient than some direct nursing care that is based on routine and ritualistic ways of working (*see* Chapter 3).

Staff needed to feel comfortable working away from the patients. What they were undertaking needed to be seen to benefit the whole team. Discussions took place around developing the skills of delegation, prioritizing workloads and time management to enable the staff involved in the process to free up some clinical time, and not wholly to rely upon being excluded from the off-duty for a whole shift.

'It's not practical to treat all patients in the same way. What should I do if I am unable to follow the guideline?'

Individualized patient care was revisited. It became apparent that some members of the team had taken the change in clinical service to mean a complete change and not that it was building on what we already had in place.

The following statement was discussed at length. The nurses still had to feel autonomous, the guidelines were supposed to empower the nurses and not be seen to disempower:

> It must be remembered that clinical guidelines are guidelines and not tramlines and therefore must not be applied automatically – they need not always be followed. The nurse must always exercise clinical discretion. An assessment of appropriateness should be made before applying the guideline and a reasonable explanation given for not applying it. Explanations for variance should be fully documented.
>
> (Tingle, 1997a: 639)

The group also reflected upon publications from the UKCC, particularly the UKCC *Code of Professional Conduct* (UKCC, 1992b) and *Scope of Professional Practice* (UKCC, 1992a). Suddenly these publications had a meaning, staff could work with them and develop practice confidently.

'What is our level of service? We seem to have to deal with everything.'

As we began to 'put some meat on the bones' of our guidelines it became apparent that we had never defined what our service level was. Both MIUs had grown over many years. No work had ever been done indicating:

- What our service was.
- Whom it was for.
- What were the boundaries.
- Who should deliver the service.

All of these were important factors to be taken into consideration when setting up a new service. During clinical supervision sessions we had extensive debates around:

- Were we predominantly providing a first-aid service?
- How to promote self-care in the public who accessed the service.
- Accessibility of appropriate resources, i.e. medical staff, nurses, equipment and support services.
- The role of the nurse practitioner.

- Training issues.
- The grade of the nurse who should be working in the unit.

Work went ahead to provide more clarity about the purpose of the MIUs for ourselves and those using the service. We produced a philosophy for the departments; information for the public, indicating waiting times and the service we provided, was displayed. Once we had defined our service level, it became apparent that the documentation tool used to support our activity needed to be reviewed. Suddenly the seemingly small project, to develop and implement guidelines, had escalated into a complex major change resulting in spin-offs of smaller projects. We became concerned about whether we would ever achieve our original goal: to develop evidence-based guidelines for the MIUs.

Reviewing the guidelines

The guidelines were reviewed as part of the process of review of the care pathways introduced into the community hospitals. The community hospitals had developed a care pathway approach to track patients through the MIUs. These were used as an action plan for the team to ensure that the patient received the appropriate care at the appropriate time, so that cost and quality outcomes were balanced (Tingle, 1997b). The guidelines were incorporated into these, enabling staff to identify when a guideline should be used. If the guideline was not used, the care was tracked using the documented evidence available from the episode of care. If a guideline was not used, this might have been because the guideline needed reviewing, or that there simply was not a guideline to cover the presenting problem. In all instances, this allowed the guidelines to be constantly reviewed and revamped and new guidelines developed as identified.

CONCLUSION

The project resulted in the production of a handbook of clinical guidelines, but it also led to other changes and led to further practice development activities similar to the process of action research (Hart and Bond, 1995). Reflecting on the process, one of the main lessons is that while the purpose of a clinical practice development group needs to be clearly defined, such a group also needs to be open to new issues and areas for development as the project progresses. The project group's first task was to identify its purpose clearly – an important point as the remit that was first identified had to be repeatedly revisited by the group due to the other pieces of work that the project created. Members of the group, Sisters Johnson, Hardisty and Spencer, reflected that the project had enabled them to think about practice:

> The process made us think more about what we were doing in everyday practice. It made us go out and search for the evidence to underpin our guidelines and helped us realise the importance of evidence-based information in the workplace. Developing user-friendly evidence-based guidelines is a considerable skill which we have all

acquired. Today the guidelines are part of everyday practice. Everybody uses them in conjunction with the care pathways: it is now second nature. There is still work to be done. Not all of the guidelines fit everything that comes through the doors of the minor injuries unit. .... Developing the guidelines took a lot of time and effort and on the odd occasion grief. But, at the end of the day, they have proved invaluable.

(Sanderson and Gledhill, 1999:29)

Reflecting on the process used to implement the change, I feel the team involvement and the communication networks in place were the key to the success of the project (*see* Chapter 4). None of the team involved in the change had realized the implications of changing what seemed such a small area of clinical practice. That was probably due to a combination of our naivety and our not researching the service area fully.

We all felt that we had researched evidence-based nursing, managing change and 'what is a guideline'. What we failed to research fully was the clinical area in which we were intending to introduce the change. Had we researched the area first, there is a possibility that we could have identified the gaps in the service and the possible areas that would have raised concerns amongst the staff, prior to undertaking any change. Maybe we would have been ready with some of the answers, the process would have been quicker and possibly less painful, but one could argue that, as a team, we needed to go through the whole process together 'warts and all' in order that we should all learn together and grow.

What emerged at the end of the project was a handbook of guidelines under-pinned by robust evidence delivered by a group of trained nurses who had developed:

- excellent communication skills;
- a strong understanding of the role and responsibility of a trained nurse;
- an increased awareness of the ethics/legal implications of nursing.

Through the power of a robust system of clinical supervision, members of the team that emerged at the end of the project were more confident, empowered prac-titioners. They understood their role and responsibilities, not only to each other but to the general public. They understood what being accountable meant and how to work within the UKCC (1992a) *Scope of Professional Practice* and other documents from the UKCC, in order to develop themselves and their practice.

These changes in the perceptions and skills of the nurses, in my view, could never have been delivered through a modular training course. Had we not gone through this process, we may never have identified a need for such training.

The power of a robust system of clinical supervision provided not only the learn-ing ground for all of the above, but when everything seemed to be spiralling out of control, it held the process together.

And now, reflecting on the process at a much later date, it becomes obvious that implementing evidence-based guidelines into these particular clinical settings 'kick started' the process of practice development. The team became empowered and con-fident. Now they have a taste for it there is no stopping them; every aspect of clinical care is now questioned; every gap in a service is sought; every solution debated. Challenging times for those managing the process!

Key points for practice development initiatives

- Project team drawn from all areas to be involved in the project.
- Identification of a project lead with managerial responsibility or influence.
- Staff require dedicated time to participate in practice development.
- Spend time on investigating all aspects of the project.
- Involve other stakeholders and experts early in the project.
- Clearly identify the purpose of the project.
- Be open to new issues identified during the course of the project.
- Have in place a clinical supervision or other system to enable staff to debate the changes.

REFERENCES

Cullum N 1998 Evidence based nursing. *Nursing Management.* 5(3): 32–5.

Department of Health 1993 *A Vision for the Future.* HMSO, London.

Eve R, Golton I, Hodgkin P, Munro J and Musson G 1997 *Learning from FACTS. Lessons from the Framework for Appropriate Care Throughout Sheffield Project.* Occasional Paper No.97/3. ScHARR, University of Sheffield, Sheffield.

Hart E and Bond M 1995 *Action Research For Health And Social Care. A Guide To Practice.* Open University Press, Buckingham.

Houston, G 1990 *Supervision Counselling.* The Rochester Foundation, London.

Kohner N 1994 *Clinical Supervision in Practice.* King's Fund, London.

NHS Centre for Reviews and Dissemination 1996 *CRD Guidelines for Those Carrying Out or Commissioning Reviews.* CRD Report Number 4, January. NHS Centre for Reviews and Dissemination, York.

NHS Executive 1996 *Clinical Guidelines – Using Clinical Guidelines to Improve Patient Care Within the NHS.* NHS Executive, Leeds.

NHS Executive 1997 *R&D in Primary Care. National Working Group Report.* (Chair Professor D Mant). Department of Health, London.

Proctor B (1986) Supervision a cooperative exercise in accountability. In: Marken M and Payne M (Eds) 1986 *Enabling and Ensuring.* Leicester National Youth Bureau and Council for Education and Training in Youth and Community Work, Leicester.

Sanderson J and Gledhill H 1999 Guiding lights. *Nursing Times* 95(38): 28–9.

Sivakumar A and Haigh A 2000 Implementing Evidence-Based Practice (or Best Possible Practice) Through Protocols in an Accident and Emergency Department in Brent and Harrow. In: Evans D and Haines A (Eds) *Implementing Evidence-based Changes in Healthcare.* Radcliffe Medical Press, Abingdon, pp. 39–66.

Tingle J 1997a Clinical guidelines: legal and clinical risk management issues. *British Journal of Nursing* 6(11): 639–41.

Tingle J 1997b Clinical Guidelines and the Law. In: Wilson J (Ed.) *Integrated Care Management. The Path to Success?* Butterworth-Heinemann, Oxford, pp. 96–111.

Tucker L 2001 Turning Community Hospitals into Assets. In: Meads G and Meads T (Eds) *Trust in Experience. Transferable Learning for Primary Care Trusts.* Radcliffe Medical Press, Abingdon, pp. 103–119.

UKCC (United Kingdom Central Council for Nursing, Midwifery and Health Visiting) 1992a *Scope of Professional Practice.* UKCC, London.

UKCC (United Kingdom Central Council for Nursing, Midwifery and Health Visiting) 1992b *Code of Professional Conduct.* UKCC, London.

University of Leeds 1994 Implementing clinical practice guidelines: can guidelines be used to improve clinical practice? *Effective Health Care* bulletin. University of Leeds, Leeds.

Wye L and McClenahan J 2000 *Getting Better with Evidence. Experiences of Putting Evidence into Practice.* King's Fund Publishing, London.

NOTES

Note 1

The guidelines developed as part of the project described are constantly evolving as new evidence becomes available, and for that reason are not reproduced here.

8

The traffic-light lessons: A team-based participatory approach to practice development

Jo Cooke

Purpose of this chapter

- To describe the importance of a team-based approach to practice development.
- To highlight the importance of using the research literature when planning practice developments.
- To suggest a reflective participatory approach to manage the process of change involved with evidence-based practice, which includes the phases of looking, thinking and acting.
- To describe a formative evaluation approach to identify the impact of the service provided, and help plan future services
- To reflect on the outcome measures used in the project to measure impact on service users.

INTRODUCTION

The traffic-light lessons were developed by a multiprofessional team that was nurse-led. Together we designed, implemented and evaluated the programme to help develop coping strategies in young people. The programme was known as the 'traffic-light lessons' in the school where we piloted the approach because it involved getting the young people to stop and think before acting, and we used traffic lights as a symbol to illustrate each phase. The initiative was kick-started by some quality-development money, which gave us time and space to address the growing concern about suicide and self-harm behaviour in young people. The literature suggested that developing a coping-strategy programme was the best way to do this, and we used this research evidence, along with locally collected information, experiential knowledge and contextual understanding, to plan a new service. The chapter aims to share with you our learning from this process.

CHARACTERISTICS OF THE PRACTICE DEVELOPMENT

The planning and implementation of this practice development had the following key characteristics:

- Listening to what the research evidence says in order to plan what to do.
- Collecting local information to target interventions.
- Using the research evidence creatively to develop an intervention suitable to fit context and time constraints.
- Negotiating and planning appropriate action, based on 'evidence' collected.
- Working in a participatory way across the team (including user representation), acknowledging and applying the strengths of individuals to achieve a common objective.
- Evaluating the intervention and reflecting on practice, to learn from what we have done and move forward.

These characteristics are important because they shape the process of development that incorporates different types of evidence within reflective practice to produce change. The characteristics are also transferable to other contexts to help manage change.

The application of evidence into practice is a complex business, which the literature suggests should be a managed process of change, where the impact on service users should be evaluated (Le May, 1999; NHS Centre for Reviews and Dissemination, 1999). Important components of an evidence-based health service are: 'individuals and teams who can find, appraise, and use research evidence' (Muir Gray, 1997:155). Experience of projects and initiatives with aims including the use of evidence in practice highlight that practitioners who deliver the intervention should be involved with the planning process from the beginning (Dunning *et al.*, 1998; James and Smith, 1999).

The process of involvement in evidence-based practice development is also highlighted by authors who propose that facilitation (Kitson *et al.*, 1998) and participatory and inclusive approaches should be used (James and Smith, 1999). In particular, Mulhall (1999) suggests that approaches similar to those used in action research might be useful in managing and planning change. Both evidence-based practice and action research have a common theme: managing change through cycles of reflection. Hudson and Bennett (1997) highlight the following principles from the action research methodologies that might be useful when planning change in this way. The process should:

- involve all participants;
- be interactive;
- consist of stages of research and action which are agreed or negotiated;
- engage continuous feedback and dialogue with the researcher;
- set out to effect change.

The service development discussed in this chapter draws on these issues and describes a team, including a range of professionals and user representatives, to interpret the evidence locally and plan change. The participatory nature of the approach that will be described also emphasizes the 'matrix' of evidence (James and Smith, 1999) that can be used in applying research evidence into practice. Such evidence includes the reflective practice of the practitioners involved, information from the service users, and the need for locally collected information to target and plan action.

FORMATIVE EVALUATION: LEARNING AS YOU PLAN AND PROGRESS

The development also has a theme of evaluation. Authors strongly argue that the impact of evidence on practice needs to be evaluated, and call for the design and methods to suit the process (Muir Gray, 1997; Le May, 1999). The approach used in the evaluation of this programme was one of formative evaluation, which resonates with the reflective and participatory nature adopted during the whole of this practice development. Formative evaluation is one of the categories of evaluation identified by the American Evaluation Society (Robson, 1993) (*see* Chapter 5). Ovretveit (1998:43) suggests that the purpose of a formative evaluation is: 'To give information and assistance to the people who are able to make changes to an intervention so they can make improvements'.

Using this approach, the researcher works alongside the service providers and sometimes other stakeholders, giving feedback and information in order to plan and shape services. This approach is often used, as in this context, during the early developmental stage of a service (Ovretveit, 1998). The cycle of looking, thinking and acting to enhance improvement and change, mirrors the action research strategies (Stringer, 1996), and Hart and Bond (1995) and Bowling (1997) describe formative evaluation as a type of action research.

TO START AT THE BEGINNING

The window of opportunity to develop the programme was created by the availability of some regional quality funding based on a proposal written by the community trust's clinical audit department. This was motivated primarily by the *Health of the Nation* targets (Department of Health, 1992) and subsequent policy initiatives (Department of Health, 1998) aimed at reducing the number of suicides in the country. The initial proposal aimed to address the problem of suicide and self-harm by developing an education package for young people, to increase the awareness and use of mental health services during times of potential self-harm. The senior audit manager who wrote the proposal was aware that the idea of educational outreach was simply that – 'a good idea', and wanted to check out, through an examination of the literature, how to do this effectively. At this point there was very limited contact with actual health professionals engaged with young people, so input of practical advice and clinical experience was limited.

The benefit of successfully bidding for the regional quality funds was that some money was allocated to commission a literature review. This was carried out by academics at the local university. The messages from the review suggested that a different approach was needed from that described in the original proposal, and at this juncture I was asked to develop the proposal and project further in my capacity as lead research nurse of the community trust, and research fellow at the university. It was at this point that the development took a more participatory stance. I gathered together a project team of 'key' people who would add value to the interpretation of the research evidence and its application into practice.

Developing the team and programme planning

Identifying key people or stakeholders in service development is strongly supported in both the action research literature (Hart and Bond, 1995; Stringer, 1996) and the research implementation literature (Dunning *et al.*, 1998; James and Smith 1999) (*see* Chapter 4). Hart and Bond (1995) suggest that the stakeholders or key players might include management, user and carer representation, practitioners, opinion makers and purchasers. Most of these groups were included in the project group, as well as people who would help conduct the research (Table 8.1). The service user was from

Table 8.1   *A description of the team, their skills and functions within the project*

Team member	What they brought to the project	Function within project
Nurse researcher	Research skills and knowledge; evidence-based practice knowledge and facilitation, access to university facilities	Project planning, evaluation and support to practitioners
School nurse	Local knowledge of the schools within the area; experience of conducting health education in schools, links and good working relationships in local schools	Designing and conducting programme; liaison with schools
Community psychiatric nurse	Extensive experience of group work with young people who have mental health difficulties; experience of using problem-solving and coping strategies with young people	Designing and conducting programme
Senior manager within children's services	Power to allow time and money to be spent on the project; links with management of the education services	Support and time for development
User representation (from MIND)	The users' views about the development of the project	Advice
Clinical psychologist	Clinical and research experience of working with young people with mental health difficulties	Advice
Clinical audit assistant	Clerical support, data input and analysis	Identifying data for needs assessment, clerical support, data management

MIND, an organization representing mental heath service users. Each member brought not only differing perspectives to the project, but also complementary skills. The group that was formed met regularly to look, think and act on information we collected. We made progress reports throughout the project to the NHS Regional Health Authority via the local health authority, organizations which could be considered both the funders of the project and purchasers of the service.

The first project meeting aimed to establish a common goal for the group and involved the first stages of the 'looking–thinking–acting' cycle, where we made time to reflect on the messages from the initial literature search. Planning the course style and content, and the evaluation methodology, continued in subsequent meetings, and involved other cycles of 'looking, thinking and acting'.

What were the messages from the initial literature search?

The commissioned literature review explored differing approaches to tackle the problem of suicide in young people. It examined, in particular, educational suicide initiatives where young people were given information about what to do if they or their friends felt suicidal (Monach and Francis, 1997). The quality of evidence ascertained by the review was limited if we use the traditional hierarchy of evidence suggested by much of the clinical effectiveness literature (Muir Gray, 1997; Cullum and Droogan, 1999; Le May, 1999) (see Chapters 2 and 3). Designs providing the best evidence of potential outcome for an intervention with strong predictive qualities allowing for least bias include (in order of quality of evidence):

- Systematic reviews, where the body of research on a particular topic is located, appraised and synthesized systematically to obtain a reliable overview. In systematic reviews the studies that are summarized are selected for quality.
- Randomized controlled trials (RCT), where participants are randomly allocated between experimental groups whose members receive the treatment or intervention, and control groups whose members receive standard or placebo treatment, and the outcomes of the groups are compared.
- Case-controlled designs, where the experimental group are given the treatment or intervention and measures of health status are compared before and after the intervention. Comparison is made with a similar control group, although the process of assignment to experimental and control is not random, thus producing potential bias.
- Cohort designs, where measurements are taken before and after and intervention only occurs within the intervention group. No comparison is made to other groups and so it is not clear whether any changes that did occur would have done so anyway.

No systematic reviews were identified in the literature search, although an overview where many studies were reviewed systematically and selected for quality (not using Cochrane methodology above) was highlighted. Some studies followed the case-control or cohort designs, but there were very few RCTs. Most of the studies were descriptive, looking at population trends or based on a process of association rather than prediction.

Nevertheless, a clear message from the review was that suicide education initiatives often had no impact upon attitudes towards suicide (Spirito *et al.*, 1988; Shaffer *et al.*, 1991; Overholser *et al.*, 1989), and one study identified an increase in suicide rates in the intervention group (Lester, 1992). The systematic overview (Ploeg *et al.*, 1996) and another literature review (Garland and Ziger, 1993) concluded that suicide educational programmes were not effective and can even have negative affects. Young adults with negative attitudes towards themselves were unlikely to change and, more disturbingly, the discussion of suicide might actually influence some adolescents to endorse suicide as a reasonable solution to problems (Lester, 1992). This was particularly true for young men (Overholser *et al.*, 1989).

The evidence suggested that the best way to reduce suicide and work in a primary prevention manner was to focus on coping-style and problem-solving educational programmes, and this was also backed up by the experiential knowledge of the project group. The aim of such an approach is to enhance young people's life skills, their ability to identify and solve problems, and to encourage help seeking behaviour (Garland and Ziger, 1993; Ploeg *et al.*, 1996; Cole, 1998).

During the first meeting of the project group we examined the literature review and developed a shared vision of how to move the project forward. We agreed to focus on the development and implementation of a programme to increase problem solving and coping strategies by young people. This led to a second cycle of 'looking, thinking and acting'. I carried out a second literature search, and the reading was shared by the group as a whole, to identify research that would help us plan the programme. We found that a problem-solving approach to address the mental health difficulties of young people in school had been used in the USA and in Australia, with some success (Campbell and Laskey, 1991; Mann *et al.*, 1991; Forman 1993; Petersen, 1995), but there appeared to be a dearth of work undertaken in the United Kingdom. We felt, therefore, that while such evidence suggested it was important to adopt this approach for our schools, it was also necessary to include evaluation of the approach.

THE PROGRAMME DESIGN AND CONTENT

The next phase of the project was to plan (the thinking phase) and implement (the acting phase) a programme for young people. This was shaped by many factors, illustrating the 'matrix' of evidence needed to implement research into practice, specifically:

- the research literature;
- experience and knowledge within the team;
- the constraints of time and resources;
- understanding the context in which the programme will be run.

The programme that we produced was similar to the 'STOP, THINK, DO' approach described by Petersen (1995), in which each phase of problem solving is represented by a different colour of the traffic lights (Box 8.1). It also explored from whom the young people might get help, and encouraged them to assess differing options for a given situation.

> **Box 8.1 The stages of the problem-solving approach.**
>
> **STOP** (red light)
> What is the issue/problem?
> **THINK** (orange light)
>
> - What do you want to happen?
> - What can you do?
> - List four solutions.
> - What are the consequences for each solution?
>
> **DO**
> Carry out what you consider to be the best solution and (green light) review what happens.

We also agreed that the programme would be planned and carried out by the school nurse and community psychiatric nurse (CPN) within the team, but that the clinical psychologist and user representative would act as consultants around course content, style and evaluation. We agreed that I would help design the evaluation methodology, which again was debated within the team before it was carried out.

The two practitioners designed a four-lesson course to meet the time constraints of the project. They planned to use different teaching techniques, including class-room discussions, small group work and role-play, as well as more formal didactic teaching. The focus of the programme covered both attitude and skill development relating to problem solving and coping styles. Specifically it aimed to:

- Explore the young people's attitudes to differing coping styles.
- Increase and enhance skills, including problem solving techniques and getting help from others.
- Reduce non-coping strategies.

The team met many times to develop the style and content of the programme and was mindful to make it interesting and fun, as well as to focus on subjects that would seem real to young people. In particular, we listened to what the user representative had to contribute here, as well as the experiential knowledge of the practitioners, and members of the team who had children of a similar age to those to whom the pro-gramme was directed. The programme used a variety of teaching aids to make it interesting including: traffic lights; video clips; posters; card games; soap opera char-acter card games and weighing scales to make the approach more tangible. Alongside the teaching sessions, the course included assignments to practise skills in the real world.

Choosing and working with the pilot school

We decided to pilot and evaluate the programme by focusing on one school, largely due to time constraints and limited resources. This involved another cycle of look-ing, thinking and acting. The audit department worked with the data from the A&E department and selected the school that had the highest number of pupils in the city that had attended the department with self-harm behaviour within the previous year. The catchment area of this school is one of high deprivation, having a Townsend score of 10.14, indicating high levels of deprivation, with associated unemployment and poor job opportunities for young people. We decided to work with year eight pupils within this school (12–13-year-olds) because there was an increase in incidence of self-harm just after this age.

The service manager and school nurse discussed the proposed programme with the local authority and school, who were happy for the pilot to take place. The practitioners worked with the Year Head, who selected three year eight classes who he felt would benefit most from developing coping strategies. Further planning then took place with the form teachers, who helped deliver the sessions during the time-tabled personal and social education (PSE) sessions. A letter explaining the content and aims of the programme was sent to the parents/guardians of the children in the half term before it took place. Parents were invited to contact the school nurse to share any concerns or worries they had about the approach, although no parents did this.

The programme designed by the practitioners within the team was then carried out in the school over a period of a term.

Developing the evaluation design

The purpose of the evaluation was twofold. We wanted to know:

- Was the programme having the desired effect – did it produce good-enough outcomes for the young people?
- Should we continue this programme elsewhere – and if so, what have we learned to help plan the way forward?

To address these questions we had to develop a design that looked at outcomes and impact on the young people, but also used reflectivity of the practitioners around what worked and what did not, in consultation with the school.

To address the impact of the programme on the young people we decided to use a cohort design. Cohort studies involve following up a group of individuals who have had exposure to a risk factor or other intervention, to measure the impact of the intervention. Comparison may be made with the other groups (Mant and Jenkinson, 1997). Mant and Jenkinson (1997), in their discussion of cohort studies, give the example of the famous cohort study undertaken to ascertain the relationship, if any, between smoking and lung cancer in doctors. These doctors formed naturally occurring cohorts of different levels of exposure to smoking. They were followed up for 40 years and a clear relationship was demonstrated in this cohort study between smoking and lung cancer, which could not have been demonstrated using any other research design (Doll *et al.*, 1994). Other designs higher up the quality of evidence scale (RCTs, case-control designs) were ruled out because of the practice needs of the school. The Year Head was anxious that the project worked with pupils of high need and in form groups during the PSE sessions. This made random allocation of pupils impossible, and 'matching' a control group with the intervention group difficult. We therefore chose a quasi-experimental cohort design (Box 8.2).

Polit and Hungler (1997:466) define quasi-experimental designs as studies in

---

Box 8.2 Design of the cohort study

Pupils	**Intervention**	**Pupils**
Before measures		*After measures*
Coping styles	Educational programme	Coping styles
Attitudes to problem solving		Attitudes to problem solving

---

which: 'subjects cannot be randomly assigned to treatment conditions, although the researcher does manipulate the independent variable and exercises certain controls to enhance the internal validity of the results'.

The independent variable in this project was the coping strategy programme delivered to the young people. The experimental nature of the design means that we collected measurements both before and after the programme, and looked for any differences within the group over time, which could be due to the impact of the programme. But what measures should we use?

Pupil-centred measures

We debated appropriate measures to determine outcome and identify change. Although the original motivation for planning the intervention was to reduce self-harm behaviour, we agreed that we should not use this as an outcome measure for such a small group, and such a statistically rare event. We therefore focused the evaluation on the programme's objectives: namely pupil-centred changes in coping style and attitudes towards problem solving.

Coping styles were identified by using an adolescent coping scale questionnaire that had been validated on young people of 12–18 years of age (Frydenberg and Lewis, 1993). This scale comprises 19 statements that describe a possible way of managing a problem. Each pupil was then asked how often they used this approach on a five-point scale from, at one end, 'doesn't apply to me' through 'use very little' to 'use a great deal'. The instrument identifies three coping styles: problem solving, getting help from others and non-productive coping. Some examples of the items on the questionnaire and how they relate to the coping styles are given in Table 8.2.

Additionally, we measured attitudinal change by a series of Likert questions based on those used in a previous study (Mann *et al.*, 1991). These questions focused on attitudes about ownership of problems and problem-solving abilities (*see* Table 8.4 for details). The young people were asked to express their level of agreement for each statement using a five-point scale from 'strongly agree' to 'strongly disagree'.

Data collection occurred a week before and the week following completion of the four-session programme. The questionnaires were distributed by the form tutors and not the practitioners (i.e. those who had taught the sessions), to reduce bias. The response rates that we report on are an expression of the returned forms compared to the total class population ($n = 90$). This is highly likely to be an underestimate of the potential response rate that could have been achieved as, due to absenteeism and organizational difficulties in distributing the questionnaire, we found that up to a

Table 8.2   *Examples of items in the Adolescent Coping Scale*

Statement	Coping style that statement relates to
For a given problem I . . . Work at solving the problem to the best of my ability Make time for leisure activities	Problem solving
Talk to other people about my concern to help me sort it out Join with people who have the same concern	Getting help from others
Worry about what will happen to me Wish a miracle would happen	Non-productive coping styles

Source: Frydenberg and Lewis, 1993.

Table 8.3   *Response rates for fully completed sections of the questionnaire (as an expression of the class total population)*

Part of questionnaire/scale	Response rate (n)
Attitudinal questions	54% ($n = 49$)
Referring to others coping scale	53% ($n = 48$)
Non-productive coping scale	49% ($n = 44$)
Problem-solving scale	48% ($n = 43$)

third of pupils who attended the programme did not get a questionnaire. Teachers simply forgot to check that all pupils had received a form. We also found that the young people found some areas of the coping scale easier to complete than others. We, therefore, had a higher completion rate for some areas of the scale than others. The total response rates for the different parts of the fully completed questionnaire both before and after the intervention are given in Table 8.3.

We analysed the responses using a software package (SPSS for Windows) to identify any changes.

THE IMPACT OF THE PROGRAMME

Coping styles change

The results are given in Figs 8.1–8.3. There appears to be some benefit derived from the course in at least two of the coping styles, with the some young people saying that they would contact people appropriately for help rather than trying to manage on their own (referring to others, Fig. 8.1), and reducing non-productive coping styles (Fig. 8.2). However, the results for the problem-solving questions are less clear (Fig.

8.3). The use of problem solving as an approach to coping appears to have reduced. This may be due to the young people having a greater understanding about the nature of problem solving after the intervention, and so their reporting of problem solving may have changed as a consequence. With a clearer understanding, the answers given may be more accurate, but less frequent post-intervention. None of the above changes reached statistical significance.

There are limitations to the approach of reported coping styles rather than actual behaviour. A stronger approach may be to use a diary where the coping styles could

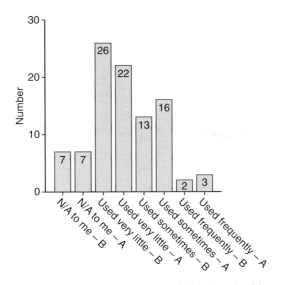

Fig. 8.1 Referring to others (n = 40). B, Before; A, after; N/A, not applicable.

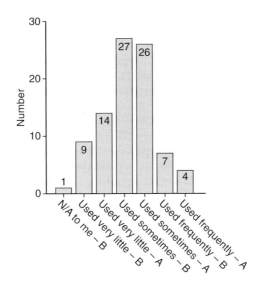

Fig. 8.2 Non-productive coping (n = 44). B, Before; A, after; N/A, not applicable.

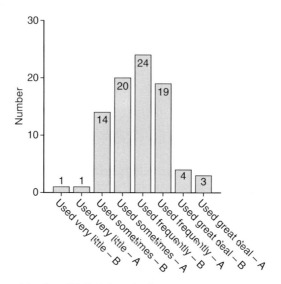

Fig. 8.3 *Problem solving (n = 43). B, Before; A, after.*

be measured using examples rather than tendencies to adapt certain styles. The limited timeframe within which this study took place also puts limitations on using this measure.

Attitudinal change

The results of all the attitudinal questions are shown in Table 8.4. A trend towards a more positive attitude was evident in all the questions asked, but this was particularly apparent around their perception of ownership of the problem, which reached statistical significance.

DISCUSSION OF PUPIL-CENTRED OUTCOMES

The sample was purposeful, based on a needs assessment, which indicated that the school would contain young people with a higher incidence of self-harm behaviour, and the Year Head's perception of classes which contained pupils of high need. The catchment area for the school shows high levels of deprivation. We know that over a half of our sample were eligible for free school meals. The school is also known to be in the lower bracket in terms of academic achievement. Also, the proportion of boys in our sample was 62 per cent. Gender differences and impact of programmes is a recurrent theme in the literature (Ploeg *et al.*, 1996; Monach and Francis, 1997). Boys often have more feelings of hopelessness, isolation and less positive attitude changes after school-based programmes, and boys seek help less than girls. We, therefore, consider that the sample is not representative of the population as a whole, but is probably biased towards attaining a poor outcome.

Table 8.4 *Results of the attitudinal section of the questionnaire*

Statement in questionnaire	% disagreement before programme ($n = 49$)	% disagreement after programme ($n = 49$)	Significance (chi-square)
Decision-making does not affect young people because they don't make important decisions	63.3	75.5	NS, P value = 0.189
Bad decisions made by others are those with which you disagree	64.6	68.8	NS, P value = 0.665
People are either good decision-makers or bad decision-makers. There is little you can do to become a good decision-maker	32.7	49.0	NS, P value = 0.100
People who take a long time when making decisions are not sure of what they want.	35.4	45.8	NS, P value = 0.299
Girls are poor decision-makers compared to boys.	73.5	77.6	NS, P value = 0.639
Important decisions affecting young people should be made by adults	59.6	78.7	Significant, P value = 0.045
Important decisions affecting young people should be made by the young person	35.4	16.7	Significant, P value = 0.036

NS = Not significant.

Greater changes were evident in attitudes rather than coping styles. This may be because coping styles need to be based on the development of skills which need practice and application. The time frame for the pilot may, therefore, be too short, and the sample size too small, to show significant differences in these skills.

The apparent reduction in problem solving as a coping strategy appears contradictory to the other findings of the project. A trend is evident that the young people were establishing more effective coping strategies, in terms of referring to others and a reduction in non-productive coping styles. These findings would, therefore, suggest that the young people were managing problems better. However, the young people may have gained a greater understanding of what problem solving is and this may have altered their perceived frequency in use of problem solving as a result of this changed definition. A longer time frame and more outcome points to measure change in skills over time would throw more light on what is happening here.

Limitations of the outcome measures chosen

The response rate of fully completed questionnaires was disappointing, although we think this was mainly due to the pupils not receiving the questionnaire in many instances. We noticed some students found the adolescent coping styles scale particularly difficult to complete, and in particular the problem-solving questions. The tool was developed in Australia and it may be that cultural differences apply to working with young people in the UK. The participants in this study were at the lower age limit of the group for whom the scale is designed and validated, and many of the young people were underachievers at school, with difficulties in reading and writing. Further work should consider other ways of capturing change for individuals who have such difficulties. This is certainly an area for more fruitful work between researchers, practitioners and young people themselves in the future.

The response rate may also reflect the level of absenteeism in the school. It can be argued that those children who do not attend school are those who are in most need of developing problem-solving and coping strategies. Further work needs to be established and evaluated to identify how to engage and work with this group.

THE WAY FORWARD

The project team met for the last time to discuss the results and to determine a dissemination strategy for the evaluation of the programme, which included writing journal articles and presentations within the community trust and at national conferences. In line with a formative evaluation approach and the looking–thinking–acting cycle, we wanted to use the results and the reflections of the project group to plan the way forward.

The team agreed that it would be beneficial to extend the programme to ten sessions, in order for the participants to have more practice in developing skills in a variety of situations. This is supported by our findings and the literature, which suggests that the acquisition of problem solving for young adults takes longer than four sessions (Petersen, 1995), and should be integral to a more long-term strategy. Certainly, the practitioners felt that the course they planned was too brief and very busy. More active involvement of the teachers in the extended programme could aid continuity. The practitioners also felt that engaging with parents of the young people and the young people themselves would add value to the programme, and they were successful in gaining a travel grant to explore this idea with the original STOP THINK DO practitioners in Australia. This illustrates how another look-ing–thinking–acting cycle has become a spin-off from the original study.

The staff in the pilot school were very eager that the programme should extend to all the year eight pupils in the next academic year, which we felt was a positive out-come in itself. The teachers noticed differences in attitude and behaviour in some of the young people. They were also pleased at how some young people who normally had difficulty engaging in classroom work were actively involved in the programme sessions. One teacher involved with the project adopted the problem-solving approach to work on other PSE topics. This suggests strategies for planning the future evaluation of the extended programme. We should plan to add more qualita-tive information to supplement the quantitative data. Young people, teachers and parents could be asked to reflect on the process and describe and illustrate change if this occurred, and should be considered as 'key' members of the evaluation process in the future.

The team manager is now working with the practitioners within the project to develop a training package to extend the programme skills to other practitioners and other schools in the area.

CONCLUSION

This chapter has described an evidence-based team approach to develop an inter-vention to address a health concern within our area. It was a multiprofessional team, which included service-user representation. The project adopted a participative approach supported by the 'research into practice' and formative evaluation litera-ture, where we planned and evaluated change using several cycles of looking–thinking–acting. It involved the members of the team pooling skills and resources to meet a common and agreed objective, and used a needs-assessment approach to target the pilot site. The evaluation helped us to understand the impact of the programme on the young people, informed us of the way forward, and pointed the practitioners to develop further cycles of looking, thinking and acting. Further developments should include working more closely with the young people them-selves and their parents. Although the project team now no longer meets, the impact on services for young people within the area continues in an extended and revised programme. The problem-solving model is being extended to address other health-promotional messages and contribute to promoting more resilient and informed young people.

Key points for practice development initiatives

- Think of developing practice through a series of reflective stages of 'looking, thinking and acting', so you can build on your learning to improve services.
- During the 'looking' phase, search the research literature. It will help you in the other phases of 'thinking and acting' when you plan what and, importantly, what not to do.
- When applying research evidence into practice, use the matrix of 'evidence' available to you, including the research literature, locally collected data, an understanding of context in which the practice takes place and the experiential knowledge of practitioners and service users.
- Use a participatory approach during practice developments. It can help to capture multiple perspectives in planning a service, which will make implementation more likely to succeed.
- Work as a team on a common, negotiated and agreed objective based on the matrix of evidence. Identify the strengths and abilities in the team and use them.
- Evaluate service developments in a way that mirrors a reflective, continual learning approach. Formative evaluation is one such methodology.

REFERENCES

Bowling A 1997 *Research Methods in Health. Investigating Health and Health Services*. Open University Press, Buckingham.

Campbell VN and Laskey KB 1991 Institutional strategy for teaching decision making in schools. In: Baron J and Brown RV (Eds) *Teaching Decision Making to Adolescents*. Lawrence Erlbaum Associates, Hillsdale NJ, pp. 297–307.

Cole DA 1998 Psychopathology of adolescent suicide: Hopelessness, coping beliefs, and depression. *Journal of Abnormal Psychology* 98: 248–55.

Cullum N and Droogan J 1999 Using research and the role of systematic reviews of the literature. In: Mulhall A and Le May A (Eds) *Nursing Research. Dissemination and Implementation*. Churchill Livingstone, Edinburgh, pp. 109–23.

Department of Health 1992 *The Health of the Nation. A Strategy for Health in England*. HMSO, London.

Department of Health 1998 *Our Healthier Nation: A Contract for Health*. Stationery Office, London.

Doll R, Peto R, Wheatley K, Gray R and Sutherland I 1994 Mortality in relation to smoking: 40 years' observations on male British doctors. *British Medical Journal* 309: 901–11.

Dunning M, Abi-Aad G, Gilbert D, Gillam S and Livett H 1998 *Turning Evidence into Everyday Practice*. King's Fund Publishing, London.

Forman SG 1993 *Coping Skills Interventions for Children and Adolescents*. Jossey-Bass, San Francisco.

Frydenberg E and Lewis R 1993 *The Adolescent Coping Scale*. Acer, Melbourne.

Garland AF and Ziger E 1993 Adolescent suicide prevention. Current research and social policy implications. *American Psychologist* 48: 169–82.

Hart E and Bond M 1995 *Action Research for Health and Social Care. A Guide to Practice.* Open University Press, Buckingham.

Hudson H and Bennett G 1997 Action research; a vehicle for change in general practice? In Pearson P and Spencer J (Eds) *Promoting Teamwork in Primary Care: A Research Based Approach.* Arnold, London, pp. 192–207.

James T and Smith P 1999 Implementing research: the practice. In Mulhall A and Le May A (Eds) *Nursing Research. Dissemination and Implementation.* Churchill Livingstone, Edinburgh.

Kitson A, Harvey G and McCormack B 1998 Enabling the implementation of evidence based practice: A conceptual framework. *Quality in Health Care* 7: 149–58.

Le May A 1999 *Evidence-based Practice.* NT monographs No 1. Nursing Times Books, London.

Lester D 1992 State initiatives in addressing youth suicide: evidence for their effectiveness. *Social Psychiatry and Psychiatric Epidemiology* 27: 75–7.

Mann L, Harmoni R and Power C 1991 The GOFER course in decision making. In: Baron J and Brown RV (Eds) *Teaching Decision Making to Adolescents.* Lawrence Erlbaum Associates, Hillsdale.

Mant J and Jenkinson C 1997 Case control and cohort studies. In: Jenkinson C (Ed.) *Assessment and Evaluation of Health and Medical Care. A Methods Text.* Open University Press, Buckingham, pp. 31–46.

Monach J and Francis C 1997 *Adolescent Suicide: A Literature Review.* Internal Report. School for Health and Related Research, University of Sheffield.

Muir Gray JA 1997 *Evidence-based Healthcare. How to Make Health Policy and Management Decisions.* Churchill Livingstone, Edinburgh.

Mulhall A 1999 Creating change in practice. In Mulhall A and Le May A (Eds) *Nursing Research. Dissemination and Implementation.* Churchill Livingstone, Edinburgh, pp. 151–75.

NHS Centre for Reviews and Dissemination 1999 Getting the evidence into practice. *Effective Health Care* bulletin 5(1). NHS Centre for Reviews and Dissemination, University of York, York.

Overholser JC, Hemstreet AH and Spirito A 1989 Suicide awareness programs in the schools: effects of gender and personal experience. *Journal of the American Academy of Child and Adolescent Psychiatry* 28: 925–30.

Ovretveit J 1998 *Evaluating Health Interventions.* Open University, Buckingham.

Petersen L 1995 STOP, THINK, DO: Improving social and learning skills for children in clinics and schools. In Henck PJG Van Bilsen, Kendall PC and Slavenburg JH (Eds). *Behavioural Approaches for Children and Adolescents: Challenges for the Next Century.* Plenum Press, New York, pp. 103–11.

Ploeg J, Ciliska D, Dobbins M, Hayward S, Thomas H and Underwood J 1996 A systematic overview of suicide prevention programs. *Canadian Journal of Public Health* 87(5): 319–24.

Polit D and Hungler BP 1997 *Essentials of Nursing Research. Methods, Appraisal and Utilisation,* 4th edn. Lippincott, Philadelphia.

Robson C 1993 *Real World Research. A Resource for Social Scientists and Practitioner-Researchers.* Blackwell, Oxford.

Shaffer D, Garland A, Vieland V, Underwood M and Busner C 1991 The impact of curriculum-based suicide prevention programs for teenagers. *Journal of the American Academy of Child and Adolescent Psychiatry* 30: 588–96.

Spirito A, Overholser J, Ashworth S, Morgan J and Benedict-Drew C 1988 Evaluation of a suicide awareness curriculum for the high school student. *Journal of the American Academy of Child and Adolescent Psychiatry* 27: 705–11.

Stringer ET 1996 *Action Research. A Handbook for Practitioners.* Sage Publications, London.

9

Capturing client voices for community development using participatory appraisal

Linda Pearson

Purpose of this chapter

- To introduce you to the participatory appraisal (PA) approach to community development.
- To outline issues around the nature of participation.
- To explore the qualities of PA facilitators and the utility of these qualities and skills for practice development.
- To present a variety of PA tools in the context of their use in studies related to health.
- To describe a community development initiative that has used PA.
- To give you a range of resource and reference material.

INTRODUCTION

Participatory rural appraisal (PRA) (*see* Note 1) can be described as a family of approaches, methods and behaviours that enable people to express and analyse the realities of their lives and conditions, to plan themselves what action to take, and to monitor and evaluate the results. Its methods have evolved from rapid rural appraisal (RRA). The difference is that PRA emphasizes processes that empower local people, whereas RRA is mainly seen as a means for outsiders to gather information. (Chambers and Blackburn, 1996:1).

Community practitioners have a strong history and tradition of working across professional and agency boundaries to provide care that meets the needs of clients within the constraints of local and national resources and political agendas. In recent times, the explicit move towards client- and family-centred care has built on these traditions and opened many opportunities for practitioners to develop new ways of working to deliver care that is orientated towards the client. Although often constrained by contracts and case loads, some community practitioners are managing to pursue local community development needs in the broadest sense (Mackereth, 1999), and others are enjoying new posts that are focused purely on community development work. This interest in community development is reflected in the establishment of the Community Development Special Interest Group (CDSIG) of the Community Practitioners and Health Visitors Association (CPHVA) (*see* Chapter 12).

There is currently an explicit requirement for care across the NHS to demonstrate partnerships with clients, families, multi-agency community groups and professions that serve the community (Department of Health, 1999, 2000) (*see* Chapter 12). The consumer voice is paramount and methods that seek to capture this voice are debated, embraced and feared to different degrees by the different parties involved.

The *Making a Difference* (Department of Health, 1999) agenda and *The NHS Plan* (Department of Health, 2000) provide opportunities for practitioners to take responsibility for areas of service provision that they are best placed to oversee, and to seek ways of developing practice in pragmatic, creative and effective ways. The use of participatory appraisal (PA) is an approach that deserves serious consideration. The potential for using this approach in health-related fields is high (IDS Participation Group, 1999) and by the end of the chapter readers will begin to identify how it might be used in their own practice.

PA is a relatively new and powerful approach to community development that can uncover grass-roots community issues faster, and in a way that other, more conventional methods do not manage to achieve (Chambers, 1994a, b). A number of important principles underpin the approach, including those of 'optimal ignorance' – not learning more than necessary, and of 'appropriate imprecision' – not measuring what need not be measured, or more accurately, than needed (Chambers, 1997:157).

PA takes on a whole community approach to development rather than focusing on individuals, or individual groups of people in isolation. This has the effect of looking for rich, deep and broad community explanations for issues that would be missed if a narrower approach were used. Community practitioners who know and are part of communities are well placed to be involved in PA as facilitators, participants and users.

The process of PA answers real questions (research), through which everyone learns (education) and from which practical solutions are generated (collective action). Therefore it shares many attributes with action research (Hart and Bond, 1995; *see* Chapters 4 and 8), although PA has different roots, is focused on development rather than research, and has the novel feature of externalizing information through the use of visual tools. Both approaches are at home in the critical theorists paradigm, or 'world view', which seeks to 'liberate meaning' from situations that are investigated (Habermas, 1986) by asking 'Why are things as they are?' The meanings uncovered can then go on to fuel change for those who have been made conscious of what has been happening in their lives and communities, generations or countries.

Visual tools are used by groups in communities to 'tell it as it is' for them (*see* Figs 9.1–9.6). This visual information is there for the group to see, question, correct, and build on in a dynamic and interactive way that facilitates ownership by group members. This interactive process is important in itself, as people learn with each other and understand issues in new ways.

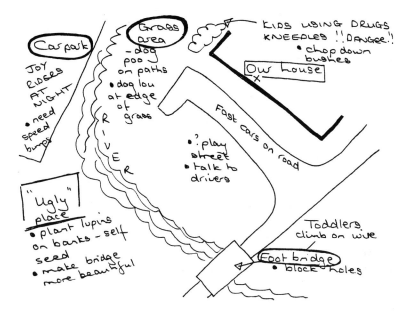

Fig. 9.1 *An example of a map drawn to identify environmental issues in an area. Maps are helpful tools and can be used early in the PA process. This one was produced during a PA training course after being asked to draw a map of where we lived, what problems there were, and what might be done about them. Maps can be used for many other purposes, for example, where people meet, which areas have resources and which don't, what our ideal place would be like, etc.*

The validity and reliability of material is important in PA studies, and various strategies are used to ensure that information is robust enough to be acted upon. These strategies include: using more than one method and source of information (triangulation); repeatedly asking 'Have we got this right?' and 'Whom should we be speaking to next?' at the end of PA sessions; seeking to understand anomalies; and accessing as many groups and individuals as are needed to get the overall picture.

THE ORIGINS AND PRACTICE OF PARTICIPATORY APPRAISAL

In many of the settings in which these methods are used, the root problem is not health, defined in a narrow way, but inequality, poverty and powerlessness. Without the commitment to empowerment and to seeing the process of change as a wider project, participation soon becomes a rather empty shell. And for pragmatic as much as political reasons, without carrying the learning process into institutions and decision-making structures, participatory methods can prove to be a first step that falters and goes no further.

(Cornwall, 1996:104)

PA (PRA) originated in the early 1990s and developed from the more extractive rapid rural appraisal (RRA) approach (Table 9.1). Early work was undertaken by individuals in non-governmental organizations (NGOs) involved in grass-roots community development work, mainly in East Africa and South Asia. People were working with communities that were powerless in some way and whose voice had previously been missed out, ignored or distorted by community planners, governments, aid agencies and multinationals. There are many parallels here with community situations in the UK.

The power and success of PA resulted in a rapid and massive expansion of its use – by 1996 over 100 countries and a variety of groups were using it, for example government departments, training institutes, aid agencies and universities (IDS policy briefing, 1996). PA networks of users, often national, had developed in at least 30 of the user countries and are used to sustain the approach for the benefit of those needing a voice in the community (*see*, for example, Sellers, 1997).

The approach spread to the UK in the late 1990s, and already includes work that focuses on community health issues. Early work in the UK used the RRA approach to focus on health needs assessments of communities (for example, Rifkin and Tabibadeh, 1990; Murray and Graham, 1995). Initiatives such as these paved the way for PA to develop. It is not difficult to imagine that the next decade could see a rapid expansion of PA use in communities in the UK if attention to people's health concerns and community development become a reality rather than rhetoric. There are signs that this may be the case. Dockery (1996) has written a balanced review of the constraints imposed by the politics of the day on true participation in elements of the NHS. Since her writing, there has been a change in government and a strong call for planners of all community and public health services to involve people in the development of their own communities (Department of Health, 2001).

Dockery (1996) challenges us to look for opportunities to use participatory methods wherever possible, even where full and true participation in the workplace is

Table 9.1   *RRA and PRA compared (from Chambers, 1997:115)*

	RRA	PRA
Major development	Late 1970s, 1980s	Late 1980s, 1990s
Major innovators in	Universities	NGOs
Main users	Aid agencies, universities	NGOs, government field organizations
Key resource earlier overlooked	Local people's knowledge	Local people's capabilities
Main innovation	Methods	Behaviour
Outsiders' mode	Eliciting	Facilitating
Objectives	Data collection	Empowerment
Main actors	Outsider	Local people
Longer-term outcomes	Plans, projects, publications and institutions	Sustainable local action

impossible. If participatory methods are used and seen to be effective, it may be easier for institutions to move towards a culture of participation.

THE NATURE AND LEVEL OF PARTICIPATION IN PARTICIPATORY RESEARCH AND DEVELOPMENT

> By bringing health professionals into communities, to learn from rather than to teach people, participatory methods open up spaces for dialogue. This experience can be humbling for health workers.
>
> (Cornwall, 1996:104)

PA is only one of a variety of methods that use the concept of participation (*see*, for example, Chapters 4, 5 and 8). This concept is a political one, in that participation requires a sharing of power. There needs to be a valuing and trust of 'the other' by the person, professional or organization that currently controls the situation, i.e. has the power. An outcome of this valuing and trust is handing over the control of power, in whatever form that power is exercised. There are many barriers to this trust and power sharing, and good PA/community development/professional training courses allow time, space and support for personal barriers to be explored and understood (Tolley and Bentley, 1996; Westerby *et al.*, 1999).

The degree to which participation takes place in participatory research and development can be seen as a spectrum. At one end, participatory research and development methods involve local people in token ways, and, at the other end (PA),

---

Box 9.1 Four evaluation projects with different levels of participation

Level 1 = Simple consultation
Young people are simply given a questionnaire at their GP surgery to fill in to say how a waiting room should be decorated.

Level 2 = More inclusive consultation
Workers use participatory visual tools to find out what users at a young people's clinic think of it. They do not feed back to the young people or involve them further.

Level 3 = Involvement in evaluation and planning
Workers ask young people, using participatory tools, their views and perceptions of sex education at school. When they realize it is not appropriate, they then ask the young people to help design a new programme, including how the information will be delivered, before implementing the changes.

Level 4 = Sustained process of evaluation and planning
Using participatory tools, nurses ask young people in several settings about their views and perceptions of a local family planning clinic. The nurses help young people identify barriers and solutions to using it and make some changes to the service which were suggested. They repeat this process regularly.

(From Westerby *et al.*, 1999:56)

learning with local people to plan and act are a focus and outcome (Cornwall, 1996). Points along the spectrum are clearly demonstrated by Westerby *et al.* (1999) (Box 9.1). Here, different levels of participation are expressed in examples of practice by describing the involvement that young people could have in planning a sexual health service. The distinction between consulting clients (at the lower end of the participation spectrum and used in levels 1 and 2) and fuller participation (in the two-way processes in levels 3 and 4) becomes clear.

THE PARTICIPATORY APPRAISAL PROCESS

PA is an approach to community development that uses the highest levels of participation wherever possible. In communities where people have had no say for years/generations, full participation may be unrealistic at first and may take a long time to happen. In communities that have become closed and suspicious of outsiders, issues relating to local sensitivities and access need to be considered (Levy, 1996).

People who are initiating the PA (facilitators) trust the ability of local people to recognise, tell, analyse, act on and evaluate their own community issues (i.e. to appraise their own situation). The process takes place when this trust is communicated through the behaviour and attitude of the facilitators in a relaxed way, using a variety of visual methods (tools) that the community members (participants) draw and use themselves.

Information is shared in an interactive and organic way between the participants themselves and with the facilitators. This attitude of facilitating rather than taking over, or controlling, is often referred to as 'handing over the stick'. This is a metaphor for handing over the pen in many UK areas, whereas in many rural areas in the 'South' (i.e. those countries in the southern part of the globe) a stick is useful to draw maps, etc. on the ground.

PA cannot succeed if the attitude of the facilitator communicates 'I know best', because participation is crucial (Cornwall and Jewkes, 1995). When reflecting on how long it has taken for the PA approach to develop, Chambers (1994a) linked this, at least in part, to the time it has taken (and is still taking) for those in the world who thought they knew best, to admit that they don't!

Readers may find that they are challenged to 'unlearn' ways of interacting with people – particularly during PA work. It can be difficult and painful for health professionals, if the 'I know best' attitude has been unconsciously internalized through personal history and preparation for professional practice. However, the pay-off comes when doing the work and seeing how effective and liberating it can be (Box 9.2).

Facilitators are therefore catalysts, facilitators and resources, rather than experts. This position reflects reality, levelling the playing field so that facilitators and participants are free to learn together throughout the whole process. Relationships and partnerships are allowed to develop, and sometimes community conflict can be uncovered for action. In many situations the process can actually be fun, and a process of discovery and action is set in motion to continue beyond the initial

---

Box 9.2 The effect that PA training and practice can have on facilitators

Non-governmental Organization (NGO) staff remarks

- After participatory social mapping: 'I have been working for eight years in this village, but I never saw it like this before'.
- After PRA practice: 'I shall never go back to questionnaires!'
- After PRA training: 'I have been trying to get this information in this village for six months, and now we have it in two afternoons'.

(Chambers, 1994b:1258)

---

enquiry. New networks of facilitators and activists develop (Sellers, 1997) and new ways of communicating and addressing community issues are learned.

Often the best facilitators are community members themselves who have had PA training alongside others interested in sustaining community development. Community practitioners involved in PA can expect to work across many boundaries, internal and external (Cresswell, 1996). Information is collected from people in the community wherever they can be accessed. The data belongs to the community, and people get involved as the process develops. It is their reality that counts. Facilitators initiate and then stand back from this process, working with more and more groups and cross-checking information by using at least four tools to explore the same issues (triangulation). Soon broad pictures of how it is for people are communicated, and how it came to be this way, how they would like it to be and how resources can be mobilized to act on initiatives or not. Often solutions come from within the community itself and do not always need more resources.

PARTICIPATORY APPRAISAL TOOLS

Although PA uses conventional sources of community information (records, census data, reports, maps, etc.), it relies heavily on visual data prepared and owned by community members. Facilitators introduce participants to suitable tools as the PA process proceeds (*see* Figs 9.1–9.6 throughout the chapter). Some tools are more suited to the earlier parts of the process to help people to tell their stories and to uncover issues, for example, time lines and maps. Other tools are more suited to analysing material and making choices, for example impact ranking diagrams (Fig. 9.2), body maps (Fig. 9.3), pie diagrams and Venn diagrams (Fig. 9.4).

Some PA practitioners are reluctant to see books of methods and tools published, so that the approach remains open, flexible and responsive to what is happening during interactions with participants (Box 9.3). The approach is constantly evolving as people bring their own experience and creativity to developing ways of helping people have their say (Motteux *et al.*, 1999).

A strength of the tools is that they are visual and use simple materials that are readily available in the study setting. Almost anything can be used to tell the 'story' –

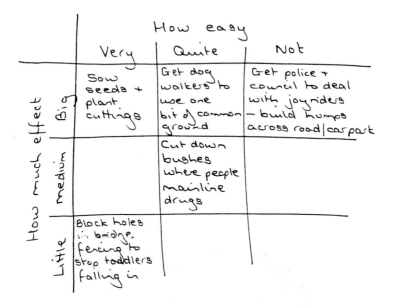

Fig. 9.2 *An example of an impact ranking to measure the impact that different actions identified in a mapping exercise (Fig. 9.1) would have on the area. This tool is one that can be used to analyse information produced earlier in the PA process. The labels of the rows and columns will reflect the type of analysis required, for example, cost, resources needed, who will be affected, how safe people will feel, etc. If 'Post-its' are used for ideas and solutions, they can be moved from box to box until they are in the most appropriate place.*

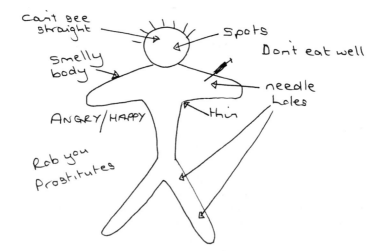

Fig. 9.3 *An example of a drawing to uncover children's understanding of the impact that drugs have on health. Body maps are familiar to nurses involved in pain control, for example. They have a variety of uses and can uncover the nature of beliefs about how the body works or is affected by the issue being discussed.*

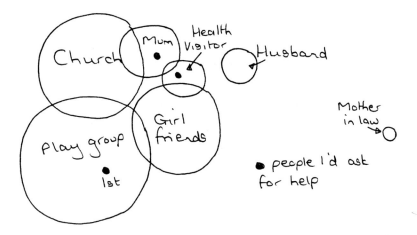

Fig. 9.4 *An example of a Venn diagram, showing a single mother's support network and the sources she would access if her child had difficulty with a health issue. This tool is useful to explore relationships between events, people, services, etc. In this example, the mother chose circle size to represent how important the sources of support are to her. The circles were positioned to reflect how her support network is linked together. The dots were placed to indicate who she would ask for advice if she had a problem with her child.*

we often use beer mats and glasses, milk jugs and sugar bowls to set the scene in a story around our tables!

In some PA situations drama is used to begin the process, particularly when the issues are complex and difficult for individuals to articulate, for example, deep-seated community violence and trauma of some kind. More commonly, the ground, sticks, chapatis and grains are used in rural settings in 'developing' countries; and, in the UK, the ground, paper, 'Post-its', sticky paper, highlighter pens, etc. are used.

Box 9.3 An example of inventing a tool to fit the situation

A simple illustration of this occurred during a PA training fieldwork session with a group of local residents in a community café. Someone said that trying to get things to change was 'like hitting your head against a brick wall'. We took this cue and asked participants to draw a wall and to name the bricks on 'Post-its'. Brick walls had not been mentioned in our training sessions! Other workers in different situations have found the concept of drawing a wall – perhaps where the brick sizes reflect the size of the problem – a useful tool. Exploring how the wall can be dismantled to the point of being able to get through it by using another tool would move the process forward. Cornwall (1997) included a problem wall and a solution tree created by primary school children in her report of a well-being needs assessment of an estate in the London area. Each leaf on the tree contains a solution to the problems that the children perceived in the area.

An outcome of this approach to materials is that the exercise can be done sponta-neously. One experienced PA facilitator shared her aim of being able to walk into any community setting and just use the facilities that are there to work through issues with local people. Another outcome is that people who find writing difficult, or who are reluctant to speak in a group, can make their input.

UK-BASED PARTICIPATORY APPRAISAL WORK THAT FOCUSES ON HEALTH

As we move into the twenty-first century, the number of reports of UK-based studies is growing, although much work in the PA field remains unpublished (Arnot, 2001). Accessing written reports is easier via PA networks because few have been published in reputable journals. This situation is likely to change as more people grow in experience and confidence in the approach, and if time is allocated to dissemination of findings in project commissioning.

The Institute of Development Studies (IDS) (*see* Chapter 12) holds over 4000 reports, articles, documents and videos about the use of PA and participatory approaches throughout the world. These can be accessed by: visiting the reading room at the IDS, contacting the reading room staff, or via the 'Participation Group' web page.

Examples of the kind of work that has been done in communities in the UK using a PA approach are given in Box 9.4.

Box 9.4 Examples of the range of PA studies in UK health-related projects

- Unemployment and health: Derbyshire (Cresswell, 1990).
- Developing a whole-community approach to teenage sexual health: Hull, Edinburgh and Walsall (Harris *et al.*, 1999).
- A participatory appraisal of domestic violence: Walsall (Garratt *et al.*, 1997).
- Participatory well-being assessment: Merton, Sutton and Wandsworth Specialist Health Promotion Service (Cornwall, 1997).
- An appraisal of perceptions of health needs of a community: Hull (Sewell and Wade, 2000).

A CASE STUDY: USER ORIENTED STRATEGIES FOR PREVENTING UNWANTED PREGNANCY IN ADOLESCENTS

This case study is unusual in that it was a large, three-centre study commissioned as part of the NHS Research and Development Programme, and it is very thorough in the description of the processes used throughout the project (Harris, *et al.*, 1999). It demonstrates how the principles of PA outlined in this chapter can be actioned and can release information that would otherwise be difficult to capture using research approaches belonging to the positivist and naturalistic paradigms, or worldviews, which seek either to control, or to understand the focus of study, respectively (Habermas, 1986).

The study took place in areas of Hull, Edinburgh and Walsall, three areas with high teenage pregnancy rates. The sites chosen were different culturally and in terms of multi-agency working. A PA, community-based approach was chosen to capture the broad environmental issues (for example, economic, psychosocial and educational) that are thought to play a part in teenagers becoming pregnant. A study that located the problem in the teenage mothers would have missed these issues and therefore provided an incomplete understanding.

The study aims were:

- to identify barriers to improving adolescent sexual health;
- to involve the community in making recommendations for addressing these barriers;
- to engage local people in working with health and family planning services, schools, youth services, voluntary and community organizations to implement recommendations.

The PA process used in this study is described in steps below. These steps, together with the tools described in Box 9.5, illustrate many of the issues raised in the chapter so far.

Project steps (from Harris et al., 1999:17)

Step 1: Project initiation

Initiate the project by identifying potential participants, identifying all relevant settings, and gaining entry to people and settings.

Step 2: Developing relationships

Develop relationships with local workers, young people and parents, to:

- promote the project locally;
- obtain background information for the appraisal;
- identify additional sources of information to complement the appraisal;
- demonstrate participatory appraisal tools and techniques;
- identify workers, young people and parents interested in PA training.

Step 3: Providing training

Provide PA training for local people, to:

- demystify the approach;
- facilitate the formation of PA networks;
- promote collaborative working between workers and local residents;
- develop a pool of volunteers and sessional workers to assist with the appraisal;
- facilitate access to young people, particularly those who were difficult to reach.

Step 4: Facilitating appraisal

Facilitate a PA of teenage sexual health in each site, in order to:

- find out whether young teenage pregnancy is a 'problem' for local people;
- get young people's perceptions of the availability of formal or informal services;
- obtain suggestions for improving formal or informal services;
- find out what influences teenagers' decisions about sex, contraception, pregnancy and termination;
- raise adults' awareness of young people's perceptions and concerns;
- change attitudes to young people's participation and to young people themselves.

Step 5: Verifying the findings

Verify the perceptions and analysis of the local situation with participants, to:

- make sure the appraisal reflects accurately the diversity of opinion in each site;
- check out whether all groups have been well represented;
- ensure that all suggestions for improving teenage sexual health have been collected;
- promote local ownership of the project;
- provide a wider debate about sexual health issues for young people;
- keep commissioners and providers informed about local perceptions throughout the project.

Step 6: Taking action

Assist local people to set up participatory working groups, to:

- agree criteria for prioritizing the interventions that were suggested during the appraisal;
- plan and implement interventions;
- promote sustained action for long-term improvements in adolescent sexual health.

Step 7: Analysing the process and the results

Compare the process and findings from the three sites, to:

- develop methods for obtaining information on the needs and views of young people;
- highlight the appropriate and sensitive methods for evaluating provision of sexual health information;
- provide information for commissioning effective adolescent sexual health services and interventions;
- construct a framework for communication between purchasers, providers and local people;
- understand factors that influence young people's decision-making about health.

A whole variety of tools were used throughout the study for different purposes and with different groups of people (Box 9.5). Over 2700 people were involved in conducting and participating in the PA, including 218 parents, 681 workers and 1867

Box 9.5 Example of the range of tools that were used for different purposes in the project

1. **Mapping** – where young people can go to buy condoms; get free condoms; get other forms of contraception; get information about sexual health; where young people meet and so on. Body mapping was used to look at young people's understanding of how contraception works.
2. **Time lines** – to explore how young people spend their time; sequence of events when accessing services; formal and informal sex education along a life line; 'ideal' sex education time lines; planning interventions.
3. **Trend lines** – to explore trends over time to illustrate a historical context or to evaluate a process; to show annual variations in service provision, sexual activity, contraceptive use, etc.
4. **Force field analysis** – to explore factors supporting young people's access to sexual health services and information and those factors limiting this access.
5. **Drawing** – 'ideal' sexual health services; attitudes of young people, service providers and parents; the differences between a pregnant and non-pregnant young woman; different types of contraception; posters to give sexual health messages and information to other young people.
6. **Evaluation wheel** – to develop criteria for leaflets, service provision, sex education, etc., and evaluate them based on these criteria.
7. **Pie charts** – to explore perceptions of proportions of young people using different types of contraception/not using contraception; perceptions of proportions of young people in the area becoming pregnant, getting jobs; proportionate allocation of resources to different types of service provision.
8. **Flow diagrams** – of choices available to young people on leaving school; of the progression of sexual relationships; of finding out about and accessing different services; and of what to do if someone thinks they may be pregnant.
9. **Causal impact diagrams** – to look at good practice in providing services to young people; having sex under 16; young teenage pregnancy; why young men don't use condoms.
10. **Venn diagrams** – to look at relationships between different services; importance of different service provision to different types of young people; influences on young people's decision making, their importance and how they relate to one another.
11. **Spider diagrams** – spider diagrams to explore issues in relationships; highlight barriers to service use/access to information about sexual health.
12. **Matrix ranking** – to rank services according to young people's criteria; to rank contraception according to young people's criteria; to rank types of information perceived to be necessary at different ages.
13. **Pairwise ranking** – to prioritize barriers to accessing and providing sexual health services; to prioritize 'solutions' to barriers; to look at preferences for contraception.
14. **Impact ranking** – to analyse 'solutions' or interventions to address barriers to improving teenage sexual health according to how feasible they may be; how effective they may be at addressing the problem; how easy they would be to implement; how much participation young people would have in their implementation; how sustainable they may be; how much agency/community collaboration they may require.
15. **Role play** – to explore condom negotiation; attitudes towards service providers and young people.
16. **Story with a gap** – to discuss particular situations a young person may find themselves in and look at the various options available.

(From Harris *et al.*, 1999:59)

young people (most were under 20 years old and half were boys – those over 20 were using family planning services).

The outcomes of the research included 31 action strategies to make information and contraceptive services more accessible and relevant for young people – these were implemented with minimal resources. As in other PA work, the effect of having done PA in the communities is left behind and other outcomes continue to be generated, some through the networks created in the three sites and now functioning independently of the project. Significant local change has occurred through involving a wide range of local people in researching other community issues, for example, domestic violence, drugs, young people's empowerment, homelessness, older people, service provision on local estates, crime and social regeneration.

Sixteen factors are identified in the project summary as contributing to teenage pregnancy, and seven major recommendations are listed. The first major recommendation is that parents, health workers, teachers, youth workers, and other community members need to create non-judgemental environments where young people feel free to discuss their concerns. Others include the need to establish holistic services, which provide sexual health information as one of a number of areas addressing adolescent concerns – these being advertised where young people go and accessible within the constraints of school days.

THE POTENTIAL OF PARTICIPATORY APPRAISAL

This is an exciting time to be involved in community development, and community development surely has to be about health. Indeed, development of communities is seen as the basic building block for the 'Health for All in the Twenty-First Century' policy. In Europe one of the four strategies to be used to achieve this goal requires: 'a participatory health development process that involves relevant partners for health, at all levels – home, school and work-site, local community and country – and that promotes joint decision-making, implementation and accountability' (WHO, 1999:4). Opportunities for readers to be involved in effective development strategies at grass-roots level are likely to increase. The PA approach to community development has a strong history and is respectful of the stories that make up community life, and the ability of community members to act responsibly and appropriately to address needs. Community practitioners could make effective use of the PA approach in a variety of settings and ways that increase users' participation. Thinking twice about how to involve people in designing services could pay off richly and might avoid the frustration that many practitioners feel when, for example, they organize sessions for groups that are subsequently poorly attended.

Training courses in PA give people the opportunity to work alongside others in a supportive environment so that personal challenges and barriers to 'handing over the stick' can be explored. Training is provided by PA facilitators – experienced PA practitioners who can now offer training and support to others interested in becoming PA practitioners. Opportunities to be involved in large community projects may be limited in the short term, but smaller-scale local projects, with the support of PA and other networks, can provide valuable experience after PA training. Figure 9.5 illustrates the types of activities undertaken during a PA training course.

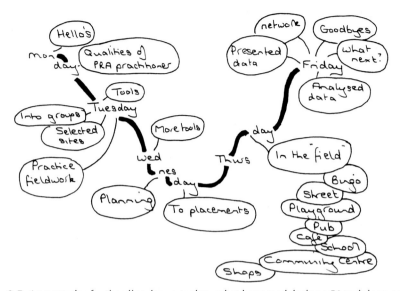

Fig. 9.5 *An example of a time line drawn to show what happened during a PA training week and to reflect the mood of the group during the week. Time lines are a good starting point in the PA process. This one might come from the group being asked: 'What happened during your PA course? Can you draw it for us?' The line could then be interviewed. Question: 'Why did the dips occur on Monday and Wednesday?' Answer: 'On Monday we realized that we'd have to work on our facilitator skills. On Wednesday we were really unsure of how we would manage the field work – everything was so new to us.' Question: 'What happened on Thursday to make the group feel so good?' Answer: 'We were using the tools in many places and could see how they worked and how much useful information came from using them.'*

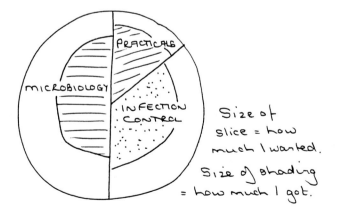

Fig. 9.6 *An example of an evaluation wheel to identify what students expected from a course and the extent to which their expectations were met. This tool can generate a lot of information very quickly. It is quite adaptable, for example, the size of the slice of pie can be chosen to reflect the importance of the issue, the number of slices can be pre-set or left open, and a score can be attributed to how well an issue has been covered.*

Dockery (1996) highlighted the need to look for opportunities to affect the culture of organizations through the use of PAs. One example of how an element of the approach can be incorporated into a university setting is given in Fig. 9.6. Here I use an evaluation wheel, alongside a standard organizational evaluation form, to access information about students' expectations and experiences of taught modules. Using the PA approach in small ways, within the constraints of work, gives the opportunity to participate with students on more equal terms. Readers will identify their own ways of using PA to contribute to their own communities and workplaces.

CONCLUSION

PA has a lot of power and potential to contribute to a primary health care-led NHS. It is relatively new in the UK and this gives us the opportunity to ensure that it is used appropriately, and gains positive evaluation from communities. The approach has potential to give some practitioners, who work to facilitate community development, a broad framework to work within. Many of the methods and processes used might be equally effective in involving staff in practice and service development activities.

PA is not for everyone or for every situation, and it does have its critics (Cooke and Kothari, 2001). However, the approach is already being used in work that has a health focus in communities, and community practitioners would benefit from being involved with this work. The approach tends to draw people to itself. If you are beginning to see how you may be able to use the approach in your own work, then Chapter 12 will provide further information.

Key points for practice development initiatives

- PA is an interactive, dynamic, self-sustaining approach concerned with tackling real community issues with those communities.
- The approach fosters a new way of seeing people, 'problems' and 'solutions'.
- The lessons of PA regarding participation and empowerment are transferable to the wider practice-development agenda.
- The use of different tools within a framework of valuing and trusting 'the other' enables the exploration of the real meanings of people's situations.
- Elements of the approach can be used by individuals to affect practice at the point of delivery, and to plan and evaluate services.
- The culture of organizations can be challenged and changed through the use of participatory approaches.
- Training is required in the use of the PA approach, which may involve some unlearning of past understandings of our relationship with communities.
- Community practitioners may be ideally placed to link with, and catalyse, community development activities based on the PA approach.

ACKNOWLEDGEMENTS

Many people have contributed in some way to the production of this chapter, particularly those working with the organizations cited in the text. Thanks also to members of the Hull and East Yorkshire PRA network, and to those who helped by who they are, what they do, and how they do it!

REFERENCES

Arnot C 2001 Diet pep talks. *Guardian Society* 25 July: 5.

Chambers R 1994a The origins and practice of participatory rural appraisal. *World Development* 22(7): 953–69.

Chambers R 1994b Participatory Rural Appraisal (PRA): Analysis of experience. *World Development* 22(9): 1253–68.

Chambers R 1997 *Whose Reality Counts?–- Putting the First Last.* IntermediateTechnology Publications, London.

Chambers R and Blackburn J 1996 *The Power of Participation: PRA and Policy.* IDS policy briefing. Institute of Development Studies, University of Sussex, Brighton.

Cooke B and Kothari U (Eds) 2001 *Participation – The New Tyranny?* Zed Books Ltd, London.

Cornwall A 1996 Towards participatory practice: participatory rural appraisal (PRA) and the participatory process. In: de Koning K and Martin M (Eds) *Participatory Research in Health. Issues and Experiences.* Zed Books Ltd, London, pp. 94–107.

Cornwall A 1997 *Roundshaw Participatory Well-being Needs Assessment – Final Report.* Merton, Sutton and Wandsworth Specialist Health Promotion Service, Merton, Sutton and Wandsworth Health Authority, London, pp. 11–12.

Cornwall A and Jewkes R 1995 What is Participatory Research? *Social Science Medicine* 41(12): 1667–76.

Cresswell T 1990 *Unemployment and Health: A Study of Unemployment and How it Affects Individual Health and Family Life.* North Derbyshire Health Promotion Programme, Derbyshire.

Cresswell T 1996 Participatory appraisal in the UK urban health sector – keeping faith with perceived needs. *Development in Practice* 6(1): 16–24.

Department of Health 1999 *Making a Difference: Strengthening the Nursing, Midwifery and Health Visiting Contribution to Health and Healthcare.* Department of Health, London.

Department of Health 2000 *The NHS Plan – A Plan for Investment, a Plan for Reform.* Department of Health, London. URL: http://www.nhs.uk/nationalplan

Department of Health 2001 *Shifting the Balance of Power within the NHS – Securing Delivery.* Department of Health, London.

Dockery G 1996 Rhetoric or reality? Participatory Research in the National Health Service, UK. In: de Koning K and Martin M (Eds) 1996 *Participatory Research in Health. Issues and Experiences.* Zed Books Ltd, London, pp. 164–175.

Garratt D (compiled with the help of others) 1997 *A Participatory Appraisal of Domestic Violence – Community Perceptions and a Review of the Beechdale Project.* The Department of Public Health Medicine, The University of Hull, Hull.

Habermas J 1986 *Knowledge and Human Interests* (translated Shapiro JJ). Polity Press, Oxford.

Harris J, Hutchinson A, Sellers T and Wallman S 1999 *User Oriented Strategies for Preventing Unwanted Pregnancy in Adolescents* Final Report – NHS Research and Development Programme. The Department of Public Health Medicine, The University of Hull, Hull.

Hart E and Bond M 1995 *Action Research and Social Care – A Guide to Practice.* Open University Press, Buckingham.

IDS Policy Briefing 1996 *The Power of Participation: PRA and Policy.* Institute of Development Studies, University of Sussex, Brighton.

IDS Participation Group 1999 *Using Participatory Approaches in Health – a Topic Pack of Readings and Resources.* Institute of Development Studies, University of Sussex, Brighton.

Levy H 1996 *They Cry 'Respect!' Urban Violence and Poverty in Jamaica.* Centre for Population, Community and Social Change, University of the West Indies, Kingston, Jamaica.

Mackereth CJ 1999 *Joined up Working – Community Development in Primary Health Care.* Community Practitioners and Health Visitors Association, London, pp. 31–3.

Motteux N, Binns T, Nel E and Rowntree K 1999 Empowerment for development: taking participatory appraisal further in rural South Africa. *Development in Practice* 9(3): 261–273.

Murray SA and Graham LJC 1995 Practice based health needs assessment: use of four methods in a small neighbourhood. *British Medical Journal* 310: 1443–8.

Rifkin S and Tabibadeh I 1990 *Rapid Appraisal to assess Community Health Needs: a focus on the urban poor.* Institute of Development Studies Library, University of Sussex, Brighton.

Sellers T 1997 Building community capacity – Hull And East Yorkshire PRA Network. *Gender and Development* 5(3): 58–60.

Sewell D and Wade N 2000 *A Community Participatory Appraisal of Health Perceptions and Needs for the Thornton Estate Community, Kingston Upon Hull.* Goodwin Centre, Icehouse Road, Hull HU3 2HQ.

Tolley EE and Bentley ME 1996 Training issues for the use of participatory research methods in health. In: de Koning K and Martin M (Eds) 1996 *Participatory Research in Health. Issues and Experiences.* Zed Books Ltd, London, pp. 50–61.

Westerby M, Harris J, Sellers T and Hill T 1999 *Evaluating Sexual Health Services: A Community Approach. 'How to do it' – Suggested Process for Conducting a Participatory Evaluation of Community Sexual Health Services.* The Department of Public Health Medicine, The University of Hull, Hull.

World Health Organization 1999 *Health 21. The Health for All Policy Framework for the WHO European Region.* European Health for All Series No.6. WHO, Regional Office for Europe, Copenhagen.

BIBLIOGRAPHY

Chambers R 1994 Participatory Rural Appraisal (PRA): Challenges, potential and paradigm. *World Development* 22(10): 1437–54.

Cornwall A 1999 Introduction to PRA visualisation methods. In: *IDS Participation Group 1999 Using Participatory Approaches in Health – A Topic Pack of Readings and Resources.* Institute of Development Studies, University of Sussex, Brighton.

Mikkelsen B 1995 *Methods for Development Work and Research – A Guide for Practitioners.* Sage Publications, London.

NOTES

Note 1

Participatory rural appraisal (PRA) was the term used in early work to reflect the use of the approach in predominantly rural settings. It is becoming more common to use the term participatory appraisal (PA) for work in non-rural settings and therefore this term is used throughout the chapter. The abbreviation PRA is only used when quoting material from the early literature.

10

Nursing Development Units: A model for promoting practice development in primary care

Kate Gerrish, Joanne Dorsman, Nicki Whitfield and Jane Mischenko

Purpose of this chapter

- To review the literature on Nursing Development Units.
- To describe the Middleton NDU.
- To describe the NDU approach to practice development.

INTRODUCTION

Nursing Development Units (NDUs) first originated in the UK in the early 1980s as centres for pioneering innovative clinical nursing practice and research. Although in the intervening years NDUs have not become widespread, there has, nevertheless, been a sustained interest in this approach to practice development. Drawing upon the experiences of an established community-based NDU (Middleton Clinic, Leeds, UK), this chapter will explore the contribution that NDUs can make to practice development in primary care.

In setting the scene, we begin by examining the wider literature on the development of NDUs, their characteristics and their contribution to health care. We then move on to share our experiences of being involved in Middleton NDU. Although the NDU has undertaken a number of specific practice development initiatives, each of which could form the basis of a chapter in its own right, the intention here is to provide an overview of the unit, consider its overall approach to practice development and the ongoing challenges that it faces. The lessons learnt from our experiences will hopefully provide useful pointers for others interested in this approach to practice development.

NURSING DEVELOPMENT UNITS: THEIR CHARACTERISTICS AND PURPOSE

Since their inception approximately 20 years ago, NDUs have been credited with pioneering innovative practice development. Proponents claim that they are concerned with advancing the frontiers of nursing knowledge by undertaking research and systematic evaluation of practice development and facilitating the professional development of nurses (Salvage, 1995; Draper, 1996; Malby, 1996; Vaughan, 1998). However, although there is general agreement on these broad principles, there is a lack of clarity about the precise focus of an NDU's activity. The early prototype units established by Pearson (1983) and Wright (1992) incorporated specific briefs, to become centres of excellence through undertaking research, teaching and piloting innovative approaches to care, and they became instrumental in generating and testing new forms of care delivery which attracted not just local but also national interest. These characteristics are evident in an early definition of NDUs proposed by the Institute of Nursing at the University of Leeds:

> An NDU is a practice setting, which is recognized as being a 'test bed' or 'laboratory' for innovation, creativity and 'leading-edge' practice in the organization in which it is based and for the wider profession of nursing.

> (Institute of Nursing, 1994:4)

By the time the King's Fund introduced its Nursing Development Programme in the early 1990s, the emphasis had shifted somewhat from undertaking 'new territory' research and development work, to being an exemplar of best practice, primarily by replicating and evaluating practice development (Pearson, 1997). The original description advanced by the King's Fund encapsulates this broader definition and captures some of the essential features of an NDU (Box 10.1).

Box 10.1 King's Fund definition of an NDU

An NDU is a care setting, which aims to achieve and promote excellence in nursing. It is committed to improve patient care by maximizing the therapeutic potential of nursing; nurses working in partnership with the healthcare team in which the patient is the key member. In a climate where each person's contribution is valued and an open, questioning, supportive approach is fostered, certain activities are regarded as being essential to the unit's mission:

- offering the best possible standards of care;
- monitoring the quality of care and taking appropriate follow-up action;
- exploiting every means of improving the quality of care;
- evaluating the effects of the unit's activities on patients and staff;
- enabling nurses to develop personally and professionally;
- sharing knowledge with a wider audience.

(King's Fund Centre, 1989:1)

Other definitions place similar emphasis on the role of NDUs to 'develop nurses' in order to 'promote excellence in nursing practice' and thereby 'enhance patient care' (Wright, 1989; Neal, 1994; Salvage, 1995; Pearson, 1997). However, although NDUs appear to focus primarily on improving the care of patients, the fact that they also aim to empower nurses raises questions about the extent to which they are concerned with the professionalization of nurses (Salvage, 1992; Lorentzon, 1994). As Greenwood (1997:7) points out, by developing nurses' assertiveness, skills and confidence: 'NDUs aim to counter the silence and invisibility of nurses, the undervaluation of nursing work and the exclusion of nurses from power'. Such aspirations may run contrary to a genuine attempt to empower patients (Lorentzon, 1994).

THE HISTORY OF NURSING DEVELOPMENT UNITS IN THE UK

The duality inherent in the NDU movement to enhance both patient care and the status of nursing can perhaps best be understood by considering the historical development of NDUs. Pearson (1995) suggests that the introduction of NDUs was part of a much wider cultural change occurring in nursing in the 1960s and 1970s. The growth of university departments of nursing heralded an era in which serious attempts were made to clarify the nature of nursing practice and the contribution nursing made to the discipline of health care. A humanistic approach emphasizing the importance of the nurse–patient relationship replaced the earlier bureaucratic, managerial models of care. At the same time, the development of a feminist critique of health care began to question the subservience of a predominantly female nursing workforce to the male-dominated medical profession. The subsequent emergence of the 'new nursing' supported by the university departments appeared, on the surface, to be about enhancing patient care, but as Salvage (1992) points out, was underpinned by a strong undercurrent of professionalization. Both Pearson and Wright, who were early pioneers of the NDU movement, were products of this era, having been early graduates from a clinical master's programme at the University of Manchester.

Pearson is generally credited with establishing the first NDU in the early 1980s at a community hospital in Burford, Oxfordshire (Pearson, 1983, 1995). Burford NDU was set up with the express purpose of exploring new approaches to the delivery of nursing care, and became instrumental in pioneering the concept of 'nursing beds', where nurses assumed full responsibility for admission, care management and discharge of patients. Primary nursing was practised as originally proposed by Manthey (1980), with an individual nurse assuming responsibility for the care of designated patients over a 24-hour period and throughout their hospital stay. These principles were then transferred to an acute hospital setting in Oxford but, despite evaluation studies demonstrating the cost-effectiveness of the units (Pearson et al., 1992; Pearson, 1995), cutbacks in health authority funding and opposition from medical staff led to subsequent closure in the late 1980s (Pearson, 1995; Malby, 1996). It is interesting to note that well over a decade later the Department of Health is now revisiting the idea of nursing beds in an attempt to 'modernize' the health service (Department of Health, 1999a, 2000).

At approximately the same time as developments were occurring in Oxfordshire, Wright established the Tameside NDU in an older adult care unit at Ashton-under-Lyne. Driven by a desire to break free of the stereotypical 'Cinderella services' image of geriatric care, the unit sought to pioneer innovative care for older people. It was instrumental in displacing routinized, depersonalizing practices with patient-focused care and with establishing primary nursing on a firm footing in the UK (Wright, 1989; Malby, 1996). However, it was not until the early 1990s, when the King's Fund initially funded four 'pilot' NDUs and then, with £3.2 million from the Department of Health, subsequently established a 3-year national programme to support 30 units, that the NDU movement gained momentum (Vaughan, 1998). The aim of this initiative was to pump-prime the development of individual NDUs by allocating funding to support practice development, provide external facilitation and support for NDU teams, and facilitate networking between units. The successful NDUs, selected on the basis of eight criteria (Box 10.2), were at different stages of development and covered a variety of specialities in the acute and primary care sectors.

At the same time that the King's Fund programme was created, the Yorkshire Regional Health Authority set up an NDU programme that was subsequently managed and further developed by the Centre for the Development of Nursing Policy and Practice at the University of Leeds (Gerrish, 2001). There were two fundamental differences between the Leeds programme and that of the King's Fund. First, aspiring

Box 10.2 Criteria used by the King's Fund to endorse NDUs

1. Development of nursing

As the development of nursing is central to an NDU, clear evidence of how this is to be achieved is sought. This requires the development of a focused strategy to reach the vision to which the team is working, along with the purpose for undertaking the development work. The value orientation and beliefs of the team are required to ensure ownership of the work.

2. Clinical leadership

Strong clinical leadership is essential for the development of successful and lasting change. The leader requires considerable clinical expertise and management experience to guide and support staff through the multiple changes that will inevitably take place. The leader needs to have the confidence and the ability to share the decision-making with all the team members, mainly using a democratic leadership style.

3. Commitment from the organisation

It is widely recognized that for change to be successful it must not be attempted in isolation. Commitment to the NDU must be sought from key members of the parent organisation through the establishment of an advisory group to offer support, guidance and practice help. The organisation itself must demonstrate a climate conducive to change, showing openness, trust, effective communication and freedom from inappropriate constraints.

4. Staff participation

The successful and lasting development of practice is reliant on ownership by those involved. Coercion from senior members of the team will result in lack of commitment. Trust between staff members is essential for the development of a questioning environment where risks may be taken in relative safety.

5. Staff development

The philosophy of NDUs is to develop nursing practice through the development of nurses. Time and facilities are therefore required to enable formal and informal learning to take place and support to be given. Evidence of methods to be used to develop staff is of primary importance.

6. Evaluation

The development of quality and its measurement in healthcare is at the forefront of the health-care agenda. As different groups have interests in different aspects of quality, it is important that nurses be involved in its evaluation. However, evaluation in NDUs covers a wider brief than quality, as proof of efficiency and effectiveness are sought. NDUs have a responsibility to act on and disseminate information about their findings.

7. Finance

Evidence of current and continuing commitment of the organisation to the NDU and an indication of how the grant money is to be used is sought.

8. Equal opportunities

The King's Fund Centre is committed to equal opportunities for staff and users of health services and therefore requires some evidence of how this issue is being addressed in the unit.

(Neal, 1994:32)

NDUs did not receive any extra funding as it was argued that the transfer of innovative practice would be facilitated, and the long-term viability of the units more likely to be secured, if they operated with the same resource allocation as comparable clinical settings. Second, the Leeds programme introduced a process of accreditation. The title of NDU was formally conferred after a multidisciplinary accreditation panel incorporating practitioners, managers and higher education representatives had judged a unit's performance to be satisfactory in relation to 15 criteria (Box 10.3). Middleton NDU chose to be accredited through the University of Leeds programme.

Subsequently, the University of Leeds scheme has been extended to include Practice Development Units (PDUs). Whereas NDUs are deemed to have a uni-professional nursing focus and PDUs a multidisciplinary orientation, this differentiation is not clear-cut, as NDUs may include members of the multidisciplinary health care team (Williams, 1993). Nevertheless, the shift in emphasis does reflect a wider recognition that patients' needs may be met most effectively by collaborative working among health care professionals (Malby, 1996).

Box 10.3 Criteria for accreditation of NDUs – University of Leeds

- The unit is a defined area or team.
- The team claim ownership and accountability for the accreditation approach.
- An NDU leader is identified to lead the team in the development, evaluation and dissemination of their work.
- The team view the concept of change as a positive experience.
- The Unit embraces a culture of decentralized decision-making and staff and patient empowerment.
- Each team member is involved in personal and professional development, identified in a personal development plan.
- The process for disseminating evaluated practices, both within the organisation and externally, is included within a business plan.
- The Unit operates within baseline resources comparable to other care settings within the organisation to enable transferability of developments.
- The Unit's business plan identifies the resource requirements to achieve accreditation, in terms of time, expertise and financial support.
- Developments are evaluated in terms of their impact on the patient, organisation and staff.
- A research-based approach to practice is developed which includes a spirit of enquiry, the application of research and participation in research activity.
- The Unit collaborates with higher education to formulate theory and develop staff.
- The multidisciplinary team is fully involved to ensure that resources are managed efficiently and effectively and to enable developments.
- The Unit acts as an agent of change within the organisation, the region and nationally, publicising its success to promote the value of best practice.
- A Steering Group, which reflects the professional and client group of the unit, is established to provide support and guidance.

(Institute of Nursing, 1994)

The contribution of NDUs to health care

The growth in the number of NDUs in the early 1990s was accompanied by an abundance of publications in professional journals applauding the merits of NDUs as a means of enhancing patient care, developing nursing practice and facilitating the professional development of nurses (Wright, 1989; Mangan, 1992; Vaughan, 1992; Wright, 1992; Neal, 1994), and providing descriptive accounts of some of the innovative work undertaken (Alderman, 1989; Williams, 1993; Lloyd, 1995; Page, 1995; King's Fund Development Centre, 1996; Keatinge and Scarfe, 1998). However, despite considerable interest in NDUs, there has been comparatively little research evaluating their contribution to health care (Draper, 1996).

Apart from a substantive evaluation of the King's Fund programme (Christian and Redfern, 1996; Redfern et al., 1997; Christian and Norman, 1998; Redfern and Murrells, 1998; Redfern and Stevens, 1998) and an evaluation the University of Leeds scheme (Gerrish, 2000, 2001), other studies examining the achievements of NDUs have focused on specific units and particular nursing developments (Pearson et al.,

1989, 1992; Black, 1993; Turner-Shaw and Bosanquet, 1993; Williams, 1993; Cole and Vaughan, 1994; Griffiths and Evans, 1995). The shortfall in rigorous evaluation of NDUs can be attributed primarily to the lack of funding available to support such work. Despite the Department of Health allocating substantial funds to support the development of the King's Fund NDU programme, no funding was made available for evaluation until 2 years after the programme was established. This meant that it was too late for baseline data to be collected on each unit and for prospective data to be collected on developmental processes. Although an attempt was subsequently made to match established NDUs with comparative non-NDU settings, the researchers acknowledge the weaknesses of this design. Similarly, Gerrish's (2000, 2001) evaluation of six NDUs accredited by the University of Leeds was limited to considering the NDUs at a particular point of their development.

Nevertheless, there is evidence to suggest that NDUs do provide some benefits, especially in relation to the nursing staff. NDUs have led to increased staff satisfaction and reduced staff turnover (Black, 1993; Turner-Shaw and Bosanquet, 1993; Cole and Vaughan, 1994), although Redfern *et al.* (1997) noted that long-term staff sickness was higher in NDUs than in comparable non-NDU settings. Moreover, although NDUs undertook more small-scale research, dissemination and networking activity than comparison units, audit and formal staff development opportunities were not enhanced (Pearson, 1997; Redfern *et al.*, 1997; Redfern and Murrells, 1998).

The claim that NDUs have a beneficial impact on patient well-being is not as yet substantiated (Bond, 1998; Gerrish, 2001). Although there is some evidence that NDUs have resulted in greater patient satisfaction with nursing care (Pearson *et al.*, 1989; Pearson *et al.*, 1992), enhanced patient independence in respect of activities of living (Pearson *et al.*, 1992), increased patient compliance with care (Williams, 1993) and reduced length of patient stay (Black, 1993; Turner-Shaw and Bosanquet, 1993; Cole and Vaughan, 1994), they have yet to demonstrate fully their effectiveness in terms of patient outcomes (Draper, 1996; Redfern *et al.*, 1997; Bond, 1998; Gerrish, 2001). It is within the context of this broader understanding of NDUs that we now focus on the work of Middleton NDU.

MIDDLETON NURSING DEVELOPMENT UNIT: THE LOCAL CONTEXT

Middleton NDU was formed in 1993 from a team of district nurses and health visitors attached to a group general practice serving a practice population of approximately 13 000 and a smaller single-handed practice with a population of 2300. The members of the NDU provide nursing services to this combined population of 15 300 people. Reports on the activities of the NDU are provided on a regular basis to the GPs and the wider practice teams. It is located in an area of Leeds with high levels of socio-economic deprivation. The majority of the population live in run-down council-owned property, although there has been a recent attempt to regenerate the area by building new, privately owned homes. Unemployment is high, with a substantial proportion of the local community dependent on state benefits for their income. The use of illegal drugs and associated crime is increasing in the area, especially among young people.

Table 10.1   *Membership of the core NDU team*

Membership of the Core NDU Team	Number
District nurses	2
Community nurses	4
Health visitors	5
Nursery nurse	1
Support worker (B grade)	1
Speech and language therapist	1
Administrative/secretarial staff	2
Total	16

The link between poverty and ill-health (Townsend and Davidson, 1982; Acheson, 1998) is well illustrated in the morbidity and mortality statistics for Middleton. The standard mortality ratio for coronary heart disease, the infant mortality rate, the incidence of teenage pregnancy and of suicide and self-inflicted injury among young people are all high (Leeds Health for All, 1994). The fact that these local health concerns mirror those identified in the government's current public health agenda (Department of Health, 1999b) presents some considerable challenges for the NDU, and later in the chapter examples will be given of specific initiatives we have taken forward in an attempt to address these issues.

The title 'Nursing Development Unit' masks our commitment to multidisciplinary working. Although the team comprises primarily district nurses and health visitors, a nursery nurse, speech and language therapist and secretarial staff are core members (Table 10.1). In addition, the core team is complemented by an extended network of health care practitioners, including practice nurses, school nurses, community midwives and community psychiatric nurses, and representatives from other agencies, such as social services, education and housing, who contribute in different ways and at different times to the work of the unit. From initially having one clinical leader, we have developed a model of joint clinical leadership, whereby a district nurse and a health visitor share the responsibility for providing direction and facilitating the work of the unit.

Whereas some NDUs have sought to impact on nursing nationally, we have always had the needs of the local community as our prime concern. The initial aims of the unit, which still remain pertinent, are shown in Box 10.4. However, it is important to

---

Box 10.4 The aims of the Middleton NDU

- Initiate, evaluate and disseminate innovative, research-based, client-centred practice in response to the health needs of the local community.
- Build a cohesive, multidisciplinary nursing team that functions effectively within a changing NHS.
- Utilize the skills of the team to best effect by working collaboratively both within the team and with other agencies.
- Empower staff, clients and carers.

emphasize that we do not see ourselves adopting an insular approach, and have sought to exert an influence both locally and nationally through disseminating our work. To this end, links with academic staff in higher education have assisted us with publishing our work (for example, Gerrish *et al.*, 2000; Mischenko, 2002).

Principles underpinning practice development

Several key principles (Box 10.5) underpin the aims of the NDU identified above and have been influential in guiding practice development. Each of these will be examined in turn, and examples given of how these principles have influenced the work we have undertaken.

Providing a client-orientated service

Since its inception, the NDU has sought to respond not only to the health needs of the general practice population but also to consider the needs of the wider local community. Bearing in mind the high level of socio-economic deprivation and associated ill-health in the Middleton area, we have been particularly challenged to consider how we can work most effectively with individuals and groups to affect health gain. Although we could identify health needs and sought to provide appropriate services, members of the local community were not necessarily accessing available services. There was clearly a tension between what Bradshaw (1972, cited in Robinson and Elkan, 1996) refers to as normative needs, i.e. those identified by health professionals, and the felt needs of members of the local community, in other words an individual's perceptions of his/her needs. Motivation to access services would be influenced strongly by the extent to which services were meeting the felt needs of the local community.

In attempting to resolve this tension, we seek the views of the local community about the type of services they consider appropriate. A variety of strategies have been utilized to gain a user's perspective, such as feedback from individual clients, focus groups, participatory workshops and questionnaires, depending on the type of information being sought. For example, a concern with the proportion of children at risk within the local community and recognition of the need to facilitate good parenting, led the health visitors to evaluate the service provided to new mothers and seek their views on how more effective support might be provided. A questionnaire was distributed to all new mothers seen during the previous 12-month period ($n = 80$), and the 50 per cent who responded highlighted the need for more

---

Box 10.5 Principles underpinning practice development

- Providing a client-orientated service.
- Team working.
- Working collaboratively with the local community and other agencies.
- Enabling practitioners to realize their potential.
- Adopting a systematic approach to practice development.

intensive support above and beyond the routine single postnatal visit. In response, we introduced a structured programme entitled 'Keys to Caregiving' (Barnard, 1990) that seeks to promote parents' understanding of their infant's behaviour, such as the infant's sleep and awake states and behaviour cues, with the intention of reducing maternal anxiety and encouraging responsive care. An initial evaluation has indicated that the programme has been well received, although it is too early to judge the longer-term benefits.

Team working

Effective team working is important to the success of an NDU; however, ensuring collective ownership among team members can present a challenge (Christian and Norman, 1998; Gerrish, 2001). Although the first clinical leader spearheaded the move to establish the NDU, there was a need in the early days to ensure that all members signed up. Initial reservations were gradually dispelled as we spent time exploring together the implications and potential benefits of becoming an NDU for both our client group and ourselves. Despite several changes in clinical leader and new members joining the team, commitment to the NDU remains strong. This is attributed in part to new clinical leaders having evolved from within the team and that, on an annual basis, the team takes 'time-out' to revisit our commitment to the NDU, review the unit's progress and plan for the future.

In considering how best to respond to client need, we were challenged initially to explore how we might work collaboratively to provide a more integrated service for the local community. We began by developing a shared understanding of the nature of the work undertaken by different team members. This, in turn, led us to consider areas where we might collaborate more closely and work across professional boundaries. For example, we were aware that, due to personal circumstances, many of our client group experienced difficulty in attending pre-booked appointments, so we established a 'drop-in' clinic where people presenting with a range of health needs were seen by whichever member of the team was available. This has proved extremely popular with the local community.

The clinical leader is regarded as pivotal to engendering a team spirit within an NDU, as well as providing direction to the unit's activities. Indeed, some units have collapsed when the clinical leader has moved to another post (Christian and Norman, 1998; Gerrish, 2000). Middleton NDU has experienced considerable change in clinical leadership since its inception, yet despite these changes the team has maintained its momentum in taking forward nursing developments. The initial clinical leader left fairly soon after the unit was accredited, and at that point a decision was made to develop a model of shared leadership. From the team's perspective this approach has carried a number of advantages. First, by involving both a district nurse and a health visitor it has been easier to maintain a non-partisan commitment throughout the NDU team. Second, it has provided a safeguard to ensuring stability within the unit when one of the leaders has either been promoted or taken maternity leave. Third, in recognizing the pressure that clinical leaders often experience in fulfilling their role (Christian and Norman, 1998), sharing the responsibility has eased the burden somewhat. Finally, sharing the workload associated with leadership has meant that both leaders have been able to continue a clinical commitment, which is essential to maintaining a current awareness of the needs of the local community and credibility among the team.

The successive clinical leaders have sought to create a democratic non-hierarchical culture in which the views of all members are valued and respected. The active involvement of all team members in practice development projects has provided a sense of belonging and self-worth that has been especially valued by the more junior staff. Communication between team members has been important in promoting team working. Informal channels of communication are well established and small groups of staff working on a particular project liaise closely with each other. In addition, we have established a regular weekly meeting that is attended by all those on duty.

Working collaboratively with the local community and other agencies

At first, the NDU concentrated primarily on specific nursing issues that involved core members; however, we have recognized that in order to achieve the greatest health benefits for the local population we need to work collaboratively with the local community, other health professionals outside the team, and with other agencies. Inevitably, we work closely with the general practices to which we are attached and a number of initiatives have arisen directly from the needs of the practice populations. The practice nurses employed by the GPs have elected not to become core members of the NDU because of the practicalities of meeting regularly with the team who are based some distance from the surgery. Nevertheless, they are seen as important members of the extended team and have contributed to various projects. Local community midwives and community psychiatric nurses have also joined the extended team to work on specific issues. Moreover, working across the primary–secondary care interface has been important, as an overview of a cardiac rehabilitation programme presented in Box 10.6 illustrates.

From its inception, the NDU has been concerned not just to focus on the health needs of the GP practice population, but also to consider the needs of the broader local community. As mentioned previously, consultation with users has provided helpful information on how to develop services that are more accessible and appropriate to the local community. We have also sought to establish links with other community workers and to participate in community development activities. For example, one of the community nurses represents the unit on the 'Middleton best value forum', a local council-led initiative set up to explore ways in which the local authority can deliver more integrated services in response to local needs. Forum members include representatives from statutory bodies, local residents, community workers and voluntary agencies, who collectively explore issues such as home safety for the elderly, improving the local environment, and how young people can be encouraged to take a more active role in the local community.

Enabling practitioners to realize their potential

From the outset, the NDU movement as a whole has emphasized the need to develop nurses in order that they can, in turn, develop nursing practice. Clinical leaders are seen to play a central role in providing direction for the unit and in supporting staff development. However, clinical leaders themselves have developmental needs and do

Box 10.6 The cardiac rehabilitation project

Identifying a need

Local public health data indicated a high incidence of coronary heart disease among the community in Middleton. Consultation with hospital-based cardiac rehabilitation nurses indicated that clients from this area persistently failed to take up the hospital-based cardiac rehabilitation programmes on offer.

Addressing the need

Initially the health visitors planned to undertake domiciliary visits to clients post-myocardial infarction; however, the literature identified an existing clinically validated tool (The Heart Manual Programme) which was designed to provide continuity in advice given between hospital and the community. The Heart Manual had been shown to have beneficial outcomes (Lewin et al., 1992; Linden, 1995). Funding was made available by the health authority to purchase a set of manuals.

The tool

The Heart Manual is a home-based, self-administered cardiac rehabilitation workbook with accompanying audiocassettes that takes the patient through the first 6 weeks of the rehabilitation process. It tackles common misconceptions surrounding recovery, explores cardiac risk factors and provides advice on practical issues, such as stress reduction, exercise and relaxation. Three health visitors received training in the use of the manuals.

The pilot

A convenience sample of 30 patients admitted to hospital following an acute myocardial infarction was selected. The cardiac rehabilitation nurse introduced patients to the manual during their hospital stay and the health visitors followed this up during three home visits undertaken during the first 6 weeks post-discharge. Patients completing a postal questionnaire evaluating the manual (response rate 90%) generally reported high levels of satisfaction with the manual, and the majority had made major lifestyle changes, for example, all but one of the sample had stopped smoking. Benefits of joint working between hospital and community staff were highlighted, such as increased role awareness and pooling of knowledge.

Dissemination

Following completion of the pilot, the health authority, in conjunction with the acute hospital trust and the Primary Care Group (PCG), agreed to extend the use of the manual throughout the PCG/Primary Care Trust (PCT). Two further health visitors from the locality and a practice nurse, together with three nurses from the acute trust, subsequently received training in the use of the manual. The health visitors who initiated the project are acting in an advisory capacity to the PCG/PCT and the acute trust and are giving further consideration to audit and evaluation. In addition, a new project involving the community nurses has evolved, which is looking specifically at lifestyle changes for secondary prevention.

not necessarily find it easy to fulfil their role expectations (Christian and Norman, 1998). Successive clinical leaders have benefited from involvement with the Practice Development Alliance established by the University of Leeds. The alliance brings together clinical leaders from other NDUs accredited by the university and provides valuable networking opportunities, as well as the chance to discuss shared issues of concern (*see* Chapter 12).

We have endeavoured to create a climate in which both qualified and unqualified staff have felt part of the NDU and able to contribute to practice development. Most of the initiatives taken forward have involved several members of the team and often entailed working across professional boundaries. On occasions, project work has identified skill deficits, which have been met through in-house development or supporting staff to undertake further training. In addition, several of the team have undertaken undergraduate or master's degrees and have been able to link their academic study with projects being taken forward by the NDU. However, it has not always been easy to balance the demands for staff development with the resources available.

A systematic approach to practice development

The image of an NDU being at the forefront of practice development can create an expectation that a unit should constantly be embarking on new project work. Such an expectation is, however, unrealistic and inappropriate, for a number of reasons. First, practice development needs to be planned, implemented and evaluated in a systematic manner, and this takes time to do well. Second, the strain on practitioners, especially clinical leaders, to be seen constantly to be achieving change and innovation is considerable, and this needs to be managed carefully in order to avoid burn-out (Christian and Norman, 1998). Third, practice development should be resourced adequately. Although the very first NDUs set up by Pearson and Wright and those supported by the King's Fund received pump-priming, this has generally not been the case with more recent units. Apart from a small amount of funding to provide a part-time administrative appointment, Middleton has not received any additional monies from the trust to support development work. When specific proposals for practice development are put forward, an appraisal needs to be made of whether the new work can be accommodated within existing resources or whether additional resources should be sought. In many instances, we have been able to review existing practices in order to create the capacity to take forward development work, and have been quite successful in securing small grants to support specific initiatives. Finally, it has been important to ensure that new projects, once evaluated and seen to carry benefits for patients, become incorporated into mainstream care delivery. For example, in 1994, the district nurses became aware of research identifying the benefits of four-layer compression bandaging for the treatment of venous leg ulcers. With the support of the GPs, we pioneered this approach to care at a time when more conventional treatments were normal practice. By auditing the healing time at regular intervals we were able to demonstrate the effectiveness of this treatment and it became incorporated into everyday practice. The audits also identified a need to consider measures to prevent reoccurrence of the ulcer, and we have subsequently focused on health education strategies to promote lifestyle changes and the use of compression hosiery for patients at risk (*see* Chapter 6).

It is perhaps inevitable that the potential opportunities for practice development will exceed the resources available to sustain such development (Gerrish, 2000). As a result, the NDU has had to establish mechanisms for identifying priorities and for determining whether the financial resources, professional expertise, skill mix and other requirements are available to support proposed initiatives. Potential areas for practice development are identified via the health needs profile of the local community, national and local policy agendas, feedback from clients and ideas proposed by team members. We then make a collective decision about which developments to take forward, and incorporate them into a business plan that is reviewed annually. As with the illustration of the approach to leg ulcer management given above, many projects evolve over time into new, but related, initiatives.

There have been instances, however, when we have made a conscious decision not to continue with a particular project. Although such decisions are based primarily on an evaluation of the service and a reappraisal of need, they may also be influenced by changes in the skill mix of the team, particularly if we are unable, or consider it inappropriate, to recruit staff with a similar skill set. For example, two previous health visitors, who were qualified psychiatric nurses with expertise in working with adolescents, established a clinic specifically to support adolescents with behavioural problems. The service was initially used extensively by GPs, who valued the opportunity to refer young people for whom they felt unable to provide appropriate care. However, when the two health visitors subsequently left, the remaining health visitors felt that they did not have the necessary skills to continue with the service and anticipated that it would be difficult to recruit new staff with the same specialist skills. More importantly, a review of the service highlighted a concern that several clients were being referred from one service to another, thereby delaying an appropriate referral to more specialist help. At the same time, a new service was developed by a specialist mental health team to support children with behavioural problems and their parents. The new team was able to make direct referrals to the local Child and Adolescent Mental Health Unit and so could provide more appropriate and speedy assessment and referral where necessary. A decision was made in consultation with the GPs to cease providing the clinic and to refocus the NDU's activity on preventative measures with new parents, and the 'Keys to Caregiving' project, referred to earlier, was initiated.

PUTTING THE PRINCIPLES INTO PRACTICE: ADDRESSING YOUNG PEOPLE'S SEXUAL HEALTH NEEDS

The principles underpinning practice development identified above are illustrated in the following account of the NDU's endeavours to respond to the sexual health needs of young people in the locality – an initiative that was set up by one of the health visitors but expanded to involve a number of different agencies. Recognition of the specific health needs of the local young population and their infrequent use of traditional health services underpinned our commitment to consider offering alternative services which would be more responsive to their needs (*see* Chapter 9). An analysis of local public health data compiled by the health authority, together with information from general practices, highlighted the high incidence of teenage pregnancy. Existing family planning provision was deemed inappropriate; there was no provision designed specifically for young people, and family planning clinics were offered on an irregular basis during school hours.

A review of relevant literature was undertaken in order to inform decisions on the best way forward. This included considering the systematic review on preventing and reducing the adverse effects of unintended teenage pregnancies undertaken by the NHS Centre for Reviews and Dissemination (1997); policy reports on the nature of young people's sexual health services (Hicken and Butterworth, 1996; Pearson et al., 1996; Harris et al., 1999); published examples of good practice in this field (Goudie, 1996; Smart, 1996; Duncan, 1997), and additional studies of young people's experiences of sexual health (Nelson and Quinney, 1997).

It was clear from the literature that a multi-agency, multifaceted approach was most likely to meet with success. We began by approaching the school nurse and then met with the head teacher of the local secondary school and the staff of the youth services department. Our concern for addressing young people's sexual health needs was shared and we subsequently convened a meeting of representatives from health and other voluntary and statutory agencies, to consider how we could work together. The agencies involved included social work, education, youth workers, health promotion, a local voluntary group, family planning services, local GPs and school nursing, in addition to members of the NDU. At the first meeting it was decided to establish a forum based on a community development model that would seek to promote personal and social health education and complementary services in the area (see Chapter 9).

Initially, we decided to undertake a small-scale consultation with young people at a local youth club. In response to the issues raised, we established an informal 'drop-in' clinic to provide information and advice on sexual health, contraception and pregnancy testing. The involvement of local GPs has enabled a prompt referral pathway to be created for young women needing emergency contraceptive protection. The school nurses also established a 'drop-in' clinic and expanded health promotional activities to address sexually transmitted diseases together with substance misuse. Similar health promotional work was introduced to youth clubs in the locality and this has been reinforced by a local media campaign to promote individual and community health and by input into local community and school health fairs. A review of the drop-in clinic 1 year after it was established indicated that it was being accessed widely by young people, but, despite the health promotional focus, it was being used primarily in times of crisis. This highlighted a need to think seriously about how we could provide a more proactive service.

The Middleton best value forum subsequently initiated an extensive consultation process with young people by running focus groups in local youth clubs and participatory workshops in two secondary schools. This exercise was led by one of the health visitors, but involved the school nurse, youth workers and teachers. The workshops involved approximately 235 young people between the ages of 14 and 16, and encouraged them to identify the factors that prevented them from using existing services and then to consider the characteristics of their ideal health provision. The issues raised in the workshop reflected the recommendations of national reports (Pearson et al., 1996; NHS Centre for Reviews and Dissemination, 1997), namely, the need to develop tailor-made services where confidential, non-judgemental advice and support could be obtained.

Plans to develop a more proactive service led to a successful Health Action Zone bid to establish more integrative and comprehensive provision for young people. One of the health visitors and a representative from 'South Leeds Health for All', a local voluntary agency, drew up the proposal to develop a young persons' centre which would take a broad approach to promoting health and include social and developmental opportunities for young people, in addition to building upon the existing work. A key principle underpinning the proposal is that young people will be actively involved in all aspects of the project, in order to ensure that the centre is responsive to their needs. A total of £160000 has been secured to support the project for 2 years and the team are hopeful that, by demonstrating the value of the centre through rigorous evaluation, on going funding will be forthcoming. To this end, ownership of the project is being promoted through the multi-agency Steering Group that includes membership from the PCT.

CURRENT CHALLENGES

Although we have made considerable progress in fulfilling the aims of the NDU referred to earlier, we recognize that there is still much to be achieved. As the team evolves within a constantly changing health care system and policy context, there are a number of challenges that we face on a daily basis.

Becoming more autonomous – the emergence of self-managing status

For any organization, an NDU forms an investment in terms of the potential benefits to be gained for the wider organization through the dissemination of practice development, but an NDU also requires substantial investment from the organization if it is to be successful. Financial support is seen by some to be of key importance, especially to support evaluation and dissemination activities (Wright, 1994). However, it is also suggested that NDUs should operate with the same baseline resources as other comparable settings in order to maximize the potential transferability of innovative development (Institute of Nursing, 1994). Middleton NDU has progressed with very little in the way of extra resources, and although we have made significant progress, the lack of extra funding has inevitably limited the scope of developmental and evaluation activities. However, organizational support is not restricted to material or financial resources. The need for managerial support in order to ensure the viability and sustainability of an NDU was one of the lessons learnt from the early NDUs (Malby, 1996) and some units have ceased where organizational support, especially at Trust Board level, has been withdrawn (Gerrish, 2000). But while support from senior managers is important to the overall viability of an NDU, it is middle managers who exert the most influence over the day-to-day functioning of a unit, and without their support it can be difficult for a unit to succeed (*see* Chapter 4). Middle managers are in a position to grant the unit a degree of autonomy in taking forward its plans, free up time and resources to support staff development, and act as an advocate for the unit in the wider organization (Gerrish, 2000). Certainly, middle managers have exerted an influence over the progress made by Middleton NDU. When the unit was first established there was an expectation on the part of some managers that it should become a test-bed for practice development identified by the trust. However, as we were concerned to respond to the needs of the local community, it was necessary to negotiate our primary focus of activity with managers. Subsequent managers have been supportive of the NDU becoming more autonomous and self-managing.

Long before self-managed, integrated nursing teams were proposed as a means of organizing community nursing (Audit Commission, 1999), we gradually evolved to assume more responsibility for our own practice, as middle managers adopted an increasingly hands-off approach. Initially, we began to take responsibility for exploring how we might work collaboratively in an attempt to meet the needs of the local community. This led to the evolution of more flexible cross-professional working practices. These behaviours, coupled with the strong emphasis on team-working, reflect the characteristics of a successful integrated community nursing team (Gerrish, 1999). Becoming responsible for some aspects of the community nursing budget has meant that we have been able to review skill mix and make changes in the composition of the team. For example, through reviewing the health visiting establishment, it was possible to employ a nursery nurse to support work among young families in such areas as play and stimulation, child development and parenting support.

Although our self-managing status grants more autonomy to the NDU, it creates its own challenges. Due to a lack of clarity regarding the precise role of the clinical leaders and their lack of authority within the wider organization, it can be difficult to resolve some issues that arise within the team. Clinical leaders have not had the same authority as team leaders/clinical managers to manage personnel issues such as sickness and performance. Such authority needs to be delegated by managers and the trust is only now beginning to adapt itself to be responsive to self-managed teams. It is also important that the NDU team as a whole accepts self-managing status and, through introducing a model of group supervision, we are seeking to instil an ethos of collective ownership for managerial issues to supplement our existing collective ownership of clinical practice. Having been at the forefront of this development within the trust we now find ourselves informing other teams who are in the early stages of self-management.

Although our self-managing status has enabled us to develop a degree of autonomy in determining our own direction, it has been important to recognize our interdependence with other professional groups, especially the multidisciplinary primary health care team. NDU status has inevitably contributed to our ability to develop practice free from the constraints of a traditional management hierarchy and given us confidence to collaborate with other agencies. However, the unit does not function in isolation and it has been important to secure the support of the GPs. Plans for practice development are discussed with the GPs and they contribute to the strategic direction of the unit through the Steering Group.

DEMONSTRATING THE EFFECTIVENESS OF THE NDU

In an era in which demonstrating clinical and cost effectiveness is a central concern to health care organizations, the NDU increasingly needs to consider how it can demonstrate its effectiveness (*see* Chapter 5). There are two main aspects to considering the effectiveness of NDUs. The first relates to fundamental questions about whether NDUs in general provide a clinical and cost-effective means of providing nursing services. This is a highly complex question to answer. Bearing in mind that NDUs may vary in terms of their focus, should the concern be with the effectiveness of individual NDUs in terms of meeting their own objectives, or should more generalizable criteria be used to judge the overall effectiveness of NDUs, and, if so, who determines such criteria? Redfern *et al.* (1997) attempted to tackle this problem when evaluating the King's Fund programme by identifying several criteria (such as staff development activities and publication outputs) that were then applied to both NDU and non-NDU settings, in an attempt to identify differences between the two types of setting. However, the problem in identifying suitable measurable criteria which could be applied to both types of setting, and the difficulty of adequately matching NDU and comparable non-NDU settings, meant that they were not, at the end of the day, able to demonstrate whether NDUs provided an effective means of organizing nursing or actually benefited patients.

Gerrish's evaluation of the University of Leeds programme (Gerrish, 2000, 2001) adopted a qualitative pluralistic evaluation model (Smith and Cantley, 1988) and sought to identify the criteria by which different stakeholders with an interest in NDUs judged them to be successful. Stakeholders included the NDU members, NHS managers, medical staff, education link staff and Steering Group members. The criteria derived from the stakeholders (Box 10.7) were then used to judge six NDUs accredited by the university. Although stakeholders were of the opinion that the NDUs had made considerable progress towards achieving the majority of the criteria, there was less evidence of the units achieving demonstrable client-related outcomes. Definitive answers to the question of whether NDUs provide an effective way of promoting excellence in nursing care remain unanswered.

The second issue in respect of the effectiveness of NDUs relates to questions about the performance of an individual NDU. Again, there are issues about which criteria should be used to judge the NDU. We have deliberately sought accreditation from the University of Leeds, as it provided external verification of the standards to which the unit was working. The unit was initially accredited in 1994 and has subsequently been re-accredited by the university at 2-yearly intervals. However, the criteria for accreditation (*see*, for example, the King's Fund criteria, Box 10.2) are concerned primarily with process issues, and it is up to the NDU itself to demonstrate outcomes.

Demonstrating client-related outcomes in practice development has presented us with a considerable challenge. It is difficult to attribute a change in client well-being solely to an initiative we have introduced, as a number of other variables might influence the outcome. Moreover, it has not been possible to identify a similar non-NDU setting that could be used for comparative purposes. It has been important, therefore, to consider approaches to internal evaluation of practice development. An important lesson we have learned is to consider evaluation strategies during the planning stages of a particular development. Patient satisfaction surveys have provided an important means of determining service users' perspectives. Additionally, as the earlier illustration of venous leg ulcer management indicated, clinical audit has been used both to determine the effectiveness of interventions and identify future need. However, the dilemma for us is that small-scale evaluations, however rigorously undertaken, do not produce the generalizable findings derived from large-scale research studies.

Box 10.7 Criteria for judging the success of NDUs

Achieving optimum practice

Achieving optimum practice entailed extending the boundaries of practice through undertaking leading-edge innovation and being an exemplar of best practice in respect of practice and policy development.

Providing a client-orientated service

This entailed drawing upon the client's perspective to inform practice development and integrating services to the benefit of clients.

Achieving outcomes for practice development

NDUs needed to demonstrate their effectiveness in terms of measurable outcomes.

Dissemination of innovative practice

This necessitated NDUs seeking to disseminate their work both within their own organization and in regional and national arenas.

Effective team working

The culture and ethos of the unit were crucial to its success. Commitment to the concept, respecting the contribution of different members, democratic working practices and maximising skill mix were all important.

Enabling practitioners to realise their potential

A successful NDU provided a nurturing, enabling and supportive environment for practitioners to realise their full potential.

A strategic approach to change

This necessitated the NDU responding proactively to policy development and taking a systematic approach to planning and prioritising.

Autonomous functioning

From this perspective, an NDU needed to determine its own direction while, at the same time, recognising its interdependence with other professional groups.

(Gerrish, 2001)

ENGAGING WITH THE POLICY AGENDA

As an NDU, we are increasingly aware that we are working within a policy environment in which we have the potential to influence both the development and implementation of policy at a local level. Although the primary aim of the NDU has been to respond to the needs of the people of Middleton, much of our work has wider application. Over the years we have sought to influence nursing practice throughout the trust and, although we have had some impact, we are aware that it has not been as extensive as it might have been. Part of the problem lies with the way in which our peers have viewed the NDU. We have endeavoured not to create a sense of elitism, but have tried to demonstrate that with motivation, commitment and vision, other groups of staff can undertake similar practice development. However, despite our attempts, we have encountered a degree of unwillingness on the part of some other community nurses in the trust to adopt some of our innovative work. Christian and Redfern (1996) identified similar difficulties for the King's Fund NDUs in establishing productive relationships with other clinical areas in the host organization, which then hindered effective dissemination at a local level.

However, we now believe that the creation of Primary Care Groups and Primary Care Trusts has created new opportunities for us to have an impact beyond our immediate locality. It has been particularly encouraging that our long-standing concerns to address poverty, inequalities and social exclusion are now recognized as important priorities by the government (Department of Health, 1997, 1999b; Acheson, 1998). This means that the NDU is well placed to contribute to taking forward the PCT's agenda for health improvement.

The introduction of PCTs has created new opportunities for the NDU to extend its influence beyond the immediate local community we serve. Task groups set up by our PCT are addressing a number of priority areas that reflect key health concerns that we have been working on. This not only endorses our work, but also the NDU's representation on the task groups provides a valuable means of disseminating good practice and influencing policy development. Some of our work, for example the cardiac rehabilitation programme, is now being rolled out throughout the PCT and we are optimistic that future developments will have a wider impact.

CONCLUSION

Becoming an NDU has fundamentally changed the way that we work and the contribution we make to addressing the health needs of the local population. Although we have yet to fully demonstrate the benefits of this approach to practice development in terms of positive patient outcomes, we have begun to make considerable progress through auditing our practice and evaluating developmental work. Despite working with comparable resources to primary care nurses serving similar communities, we have been able to take forward innovative practice development that has benefited the local community and had an impact on health care services more broadly. We work within the same constraints as any other group of primary care nurses: what perhaps makes us different to some is that we have managed to stand back from our everyday practice and consider how we might do things differently and improve the service we provide to the communities we serve. The fact that we have been accredited as an NDU has, we believe, helped us to gain support from key stakeholders; however, we would contend that other primary care teams could achieve similarly without necessarily becoming a Nursing or Practice Development Unit. What is essential is that they share a collective vision for developing practice in response to client need and are committed to partnership working and a multidisciplinary, multi-agency approach to service development.

As we look to the future, we recognize that riding the waves of change in health care policy, while maintaining innovation and creativity in clinical practice, will present an enormous challenge. However, with the current government's emphasis on developing primary care, we now believe that the creation of Primary Care Trusts has resulted in considerable opportunity for primary care nurses to be more proactively involved in innovative service development. From our personal experiences, we would contend that NDUs provide one model for practice development that can facilitate nurses being actively involved in this agenda.

Key points for practice development initiatives

The team

- Ensure that a clinical leader is identified to lead the team in the development, evaluation and dissemination of their work.
- Invest in team-building activities, to ensure that all members of the team are committed to the initiative.
- Develop a shared vision of how the needs of the client group served can be met most effectively by the team.
- Develop individual team members through Personal Development Plans and clinical supervision.

Support mechanisms

- Ensure support is forthcoming from both senior and middle managers.
- Develop links with higher education to assist in evaluating and disseminating practice development initiatives.
- Consider establishing a Steering Group, comprising key stakeholders who can provide support and guidance and act as advocates for the initiative within the larger organization.
- Establish networks with other teams undertaking similar practice development work.
- Consider utilizing an external accrediting body to support the development.

Practice development initiatives

- Take account of the local and national policy contexts when planning practice development initiatives.
- Develop an action plan/business plan that identifies priorities for practice development, resources required, team members' responsibilities, staff development needs, timescales, etc.

- Identify evaluation and dissemination strategies when planning project work.
- Involve all members of staff in practice development initiatives to instil ownership.
- Develop collaborative initiatives with the wider multidisciplinary team and with other agencies.

Finally, recognize that it takes TIME to succeed!

REFERENCES

Acheson SD 1998 *Independent Inquiry into Inequalities in Health*. The Stationery Office, London.

Alderman C 1989 Awaiting developments. *Nursing Standard* 4(8): 20–1.

Audit Commission 1999 *First Assessment: A Review of District Nursing Services in England and Wales*. Audit Commission, London.

Barnard KE 1990 *Keys to Caregiving Study Guide*. Nurse Child Assessment Satellite Training, Washington.

Black M 1993 *The Growth of Tameside Nursing Development Unit and Exploration of Perceived Changes in Nursing Practice Over a Ten-Year Period*. King's Fund Centre, London.

Bond S 1998 Review: Research, audit and networking activity in nursing development units. *NT Research* 3(4): 289.

Christian S and Norman I 1998 Clinical leadership in nursing development units. *Journal of Advanced Nursing* 27: 108–16.

Christian S and Redfern S 1996 Three years on: how NDUs are meeting the challenge. *Nursing Times* 92(47): 35–7.

Cole A and Vaughan B 1994 *Reflections Three Years On*. King's Fund Centre, London.

Department of Health 1997 *The New NHS: Modern, Dependable*. Department of Health, London.

Department of Health 1999a *Making a Difference: Strengthening the Nursing, Midwifery and Health Visiting Contribution to Health And Healthcare*. Department of Health, London.

Department of Health 1999b *Saving Lives: Our Healthier Nation*. Department of Health, London.

Department of Health 2000 *The NHS Plan: A Plan for Investment, A Plan for Reform*. Department of Health, London.

Draper J 1996 Nursing development units: an opportunity for evaluation. *Journal of Advanced Nursing* 23: 267–71.

Duncan C 1997 Sexual Health Fayre: what pupils thought. *Primary Health Care* 70(10): 26–8.

Gerrish K 1999 Teamwork in primary care: an evaluation of the contribution of integrated community nursing teams. *Health and Social Care in the Community* 7(5): 367–75.

Gerrish K 2000 Nursing Development Units: factors influencing their progress. *British Journal of Nursing* 9(10): 626–30.

Gerrish K 2001 A pluralistic evaluation of nursing/practice development units. *Journal of Clinical Nursing* 10(1): 109–18.

Gerrish K, Ferguson A, Kitching N and Mischenko J 2000 Developing primary care nursing: the contribution of Nursing Development Units. *Journal of Community Nursing* 14: 6, 8, 10, 14.

Goudie H 1996 Making health services more accessible to younger people. *Nursing Times* 92(24): 45–6.

Greenwood J 1997 Should nursing development units be accredited? *Collegian* 4(1): 6–11.

Griffiths P and Evans A 1995 *Evaluation of a Nursing-led, In-patient Service: An Interim Report.* King's Fund Centre, London.

Harris J, Sellers T and Wallman S 1999 *User Orientated Strategies for Preventing Unwanted Pregnancy in Adolescents.* Final report. NHS Research and Development Programme. National Research Register Reference FO 300234. NHS Executive South East, London.

Hicken I and Butterworth T 1996 *Partnerships in Sexual Health and Sex Education: A Briefing Paper.* School of Nursing, University of Manchester, Manchester.

Institute of Nursing 1994 *Nursing Development Unit Accreditation Scheme.* University of Leeds, Leeds.

Keatinge D and Scarfe C 1998 Creating a nursing development unit in a dementia care context. *International Journal of Nursing Practice* 4: 120–5.

King's Fund Centre 1989 *Nursing Development Units.* King's Fund, London.

King's Fund Development Centre 1996 Developments in hospital and community links. *Nursing Standard* 10(42): 32–3.

Leeds Health for All 1994 *Redressing the Balance: Health Inequality in Leeds.* Leeds Health Authority, Leeds.

Lewin B, Robertson I H, Cay E L, Irving J B and Campbell M 1992 A self-help post MI package – The Heart Manual, effects on psychological adjustment, hospitalisation and GP consultation. *Lancet* 339: 1036–40.

Linden B 1995 Evaluation of a home-based rehabilitation programme for patient recovery from acute myocardial infarction. *Journal of Intensive and Critical Care Nursing* 11. 10–13.

Lloyd S 1995 The independent NDU. *Nursing Times* 91(35): 30–1.

Lorentzon M 1994 Nursing development units: professionalization strategy for nurses, cheap service option or genuine improvement in patient care? (Editorial). *Journal of Advanced Nursing* 19: 835–6.

Malby R 1996 Nursing Development Units in the United Kingdom. *Advanced Practice Nursing Quarterly* 1(4): 20–7.

Mangan P 1992 Where to from here? *Nursing Times* 88(50): 34–5.

Manthey M 1980 *The Practice of Primary Nursing.* Blackwell Scientific Publications, Oxford.

Mischenko J 2002 Theoretical underpinnings of empowerment: A framework for self-managed teams. *Community Practitioner* 75(6): 218–22.

Neal K 1994 The function and aims of nursing development units. *Nursing Times* 90(41): 31–3.

Nelson M and Quinney D 1997 Evaluating a school-based health clinic. *Health Visitor* 70(11): 419–21.

NHS Centre for Reviews and Dissemination 1997 Effective health care: preventing and reducing the adverse effects of unintended teenage pregnancies. *Effective Health Care* bulletin 3(1). NHS Centre for Reviews and Dissemination, University of York, York.

Page S 1995 Practice development units: progress update. *Nursing Standard* 10(3): 25–8.

Pearson A 1983 *The Clinical Nursing Unit.* Heinemann, London.

Pearson A 1995 A history of Nursing Development Units. In: Salvage J and Wright S (Eds) *Nursing Development Units: A Force for Change.* Scutari, Harrow, pp. 27–49.

Pearson A 1997 An evaluation of the King's Fund Centre Nursing Development Unit Network 1989–91. *Journal of Clinical Nursing* 6: 25–33.

Pearson A, Durant I and Punton S 1989 Determining quality in a unit where nursing is the primary intervention. *Journal of Advanced Nursing* 14: 269–73.

Pearson A, Punton S and Durand I 1992 *Nursing Beds: An Evaluation of Therapeutic Nursing.* Scutari, London.

Pearson S, Cornah D, Diamond I, Ingham R, Peckham S and Hyde M 1996 *Promoting Young People's Sexual Health Services.* (Report commissioned by the Health Education Authority.) Brook Advisory Centre, London.

Redfern S and Murrells T 1998 Research, audit and networking activity in nursing development units. *NT Research* 3(4): 275–87.

Redfern S and Stevens W 1998 Nursing development units: their structure and orientation. *Journal of Clinical Nursing* 7: 218–26.

Redfern S, Normand C, Christian S, Gilmore A, Murrells T, Norman I and Stevens W 1997 An evaluation of nursing development units. *NT Research* 2(4): 292–303.

Robinson J and Elkan R 1996 *Health Needs Assessment: Theory and Practice.* Churchill Livingstone, Edinburgh.

Salvage J 1992 The new nursing: empowering patients or empowering nurses? In: Robinson J, Gray A and Elkan R (Eds) *Policy Issues in Nursing.* Open University Press, Buckingham, pp. 9–23.

Salvage J 1995 Greenhouses, flagships and umbrellas. In: Salvage J and Wright S (Eds) *Nursing Development Units: A Force for Change.* Scutari, London, pp. 51–74.

Smart S 1996 Addressing the health needs of teenagers with a drop-in clinic. *Nursing Standard* 10(43): 43–5.

Smith G and Cantley C 1988 Pluralistic evaluation. In: Lishman J (Ed.) *Evaluation,* 2nd edn. Jessica Kingsley, London, pp. 118–36.

Townsend P and Davidson N 1982 *Inequalities in Health: The Black Report.* Penguin, Harmondsworth.

Turner-Shaw J and Bosanquet N 1993 *Nursing Development Units: A Way to Develop Nurses and Nursing.* King's Fund Centre, London.

Vaughan B 1992 The pursuit of excellence. *Nursing Times* 88(31): 26–8.

Vaughan B 1998 The story of NDUs: How the nursing, midwifery and health visiting development unit programme began. *NT Research* 3(4): 272–4.

Williams C 1993 Practice development units: the next step? *Nursing Times* 8(11): 25–9.

Wright S 1989 Defining the Nursing Development Unit. *Nursing Standard* 4(7): 29–31.

Wright S 1992 Exporting excellence. *Nursing Times* 88(39): 40–2.

Wright S 1994 Catalysts for change. *Elderly Care* 6(3): 33.

Section 3

11

Lessons for practice development

Jane Griffiths and Rosamund Bryar

INTRODUCTION

The purpose of this concluding chapter is to draw together some of the themes that have emerged from this book and to consider the way ahead for practice development in community nursing. As discussed in Chapter 1, this is an exciting time for practice development in community nursing. For the first time nurses in clinical practice have been included on the executive boards of Primary Care Trusts (PCTs), meaning that they can have a significant impact on the service development agenda. With such influence also comes responsibility. Part of that responsibility is to ensure that each PCT becomes an environment open to and enthusiastic about change, which will improve services and outcomes for individuals, families and communities. Such enthusiasm will be reinforced for staff if they have positive experiences of the change process themselves. Such experiences may be facilitated by the ideas and methods discussed in Sections 1 and 2 of this book.

In the introductory chapter, we stated that one of our main aims was to disseminate good practice and practical ideas from practitioners and others about how you, as community nurses, might go about changing practice in primary health care. The book was presented in four sections. The first offered the theoretical underpinnings to practice development. It explored: the terms that are in everyday use, the meaning and availability of 'evidence' to support developments in practice, our understanding of the change process based on a review of approaches to change, with practical examples from different settings, and, finally, the importance of evaluating developments in practice. In the second section of the book the practical application of some of this theory was explored through the presentation of the real-life experiences of practice development in a range of different primary health care practice settings. It is hoped that elements from these examples will be applicable to practice development initiatives with which you are concerned. The final section provides a range of resources which it is anticipated will support practice development activities and facilitate sharing of knowledge regarding practice development.

Initiating change in practice is not easy. Dissemination of research findings is not a straightforward process, and utilization of those research findings does not happen automatically. We know something about the strategies that work when attempting to develop practice, services, staff and communities, or implement research in practice, but we need to explore this further, as the theory and practice presented in this book have demonstrated. It is likely that there are 'no magic bullets' as Joyce Marshall (in Chapter 6) points out: the context of care is so variable, and the make-up of teams in primary health care so unique, that there are unlikely ever to be immutable rules about how best to achieve developments in practice. However, there are guiding principles and there are certain themes that have been repeated by many of the authors in their chapters. The nature of the development may have been quite different, and the context in which it took place may have varied widely, but there are some key points.

PLANNING THE PROJECT

The first lesson is the importance of planning a project. It is perhaps tempting to rush at a project bursting with ideas and enthusiasm without properly thinking it through. The need for planning is identified in Section 1 (*see* Chapters 4 and 5) and reinforced in the examples in Section 2. For example, in Chapter 8, Jo Cooke uses the visual symbol of traffic lights to convey the importance of stopping and thinking before acting. This image was used first as a mechanism for helping vulnerable adolescents to develop problem-solving strategies, but also as an approach to carrying out a project. In Chapter 7 Hilary Gledhill, with the benefit of hindsight, acknowledges that in introducing clinical guidelines to two minor injury units, had she researched the clinical area more fully and understood the context in which the project was to take place (stop, think as Jo Cooke describes in Chapter 8), the process may have run more smoothly. Linda Pearson, in Chapter 9, emphasizes the importance of planning when working with communities using participatory appraisal. Planning a project also involves identifying at the outset any potential barriers that will need to be overcome, and strategies for achieving this. This includes, for example, the possibility of resistance from staff, which Hilary Gledhill overcame by introducing change via a system of clinical supervision.

A vitally important consideration at the planning stage is the availability of the financial and other resources needed to carry out the project successfully. Once the project lead or facilitator has been identified or appointed, it may be possible to implement the change in practice within existing resources. Kate Gerrish, Joanne Dorsman, Nicki Whitfield and Jane Mischenko in Chapter 10 found that this was possible in most cases, although they did have a small amount of funding for part-time administrative support. These authors pointed out that managing a project without additional funding is often encouraged if the project is to be diffused into mainstream practice where there will be no extra financial support. If, however, there are likely to be major expenses that may hinder the completion of the project, it is important to recognize this and ensure that the project is adequately resourced before you get started.

It is not just financial support that is important. The project also needs the support of the organization if it is to be successful (*see* Chapter 4). Kate Gerrish and colleagues found middle managers to be the most important, as they affect day-to-day functioning of Nursing Development Units (NDUs). This group pointed out that middle managers could free up time and resources, and act as an advocate for the project in the wider organization. They also emphasized the need for practitioners to be allowed to work autonomously, because clinical leaders may lack authority in the wider organization. The issues raised by this group mirror our experiences as lead professionals in the two community trusts in which we worked: the support of the organization, particularly team leaders, middle managers and the directors of nursing, was vitally important, as was the encouragement of the organization to work autonomously. Indeed, one of the strengths of Hilary Gledhill's project was that, as manager of the minor injury units, she was able to free up time for staff to attend clinical supervision sessions and work on the clinical guidelines, often within existing resources.

Another clear message from the projects was the importance of using the research literature when planning the project (*see* Chapter 3). As Jo Cooke pointed out in Chapter 8, evidence includes research literature, locally collected data, an understanding of the context in which development takes place, experiential knowledge of practitioners and service users. Further, Joyce Marshall highlighted in her analysis of the implementation of clinical guidelines in the NEBPINY project (*see* Chapter 6) that research evidence must be used in conjunction with patient priorities and preferences, and clinical judgement. The discussion in Chapter 3 and Figs 3.1 and 3.2 reinforce the practice view presented by Joyce Marshall and Jo Cooke.

THE PROCESS

A recurring message that has come from this book is that a bottom-up approach to practice development, in which the nurses who are doing the work are valued and included, is essential. This is not to suggest that nurses do not require leadership, facilitation and a certain amount of direction to find imaginative solutions to problems. Practice development is not easy and facilitation is essential, particularly in the early stages. Leadership within a project, however, is entirely different from a top-down, management-led approach, where a new initiative is imposed on staff with minimal consultation. Joyce Marshall found that staff in the primary health care teams needed to own the process of guideline implementation. The teams identified their own needs and were therefore motivated to improve practice. Jo Cooke found that it was important that all staff were involved with the planning process right from the start of the project. She comments that a participatory, inclusive approach not only motivates practitioners to change but also captures multiple perspectives, which is essential when planning and developing a service.

Another crucial aspect of the process is teamwork. The team includes everyone who helps the project to reach a successful conclusion. Teamwork involves recognizing the role and responsibilities of all team members in reaching a shared goal. All the projects emphasized the need to involve stakeholders and opinion leaders, an important aspect of the change process discussed in Chapter 4. The projects also stressed the importance of sharing skills and supporting peers within the immediate team. In Joyce Marshall's project, she analysed the characteristics of the general practice that was less successful in implementing the clinical guidelines for management of venous ulceration in the community. In this practice the skills to manage leg ulcers rested with one nurse. The other nurses tended to defer to her, rather than developing skills themselves so that the practice could work as a team.

An important aspect of team working is that the team should be democratic and non-hierarchical, which was how Kate Gerrish, Joanne Dorsman, Nicki Whitfield and Jane Mischenko described the Middleton NDU, which was committed to multi-disciplinary working.

Empowering staff and the team is clearly important, but of equal importance is empowering the client. In her description of the process and application of participatory appraisal, Linda Pearson demonstrates that such participation is central to the process. Joyce Marshall discovered the importance of presenting information to the patient to enable him or her to make an informed choice. This was key to the implementation of guidelines for managing venous leg ulcers, where 'patient non-compliance' is a problem commonly perceived by nurses. Joyce Marshall pointed out that in relation to implementing clinical guidelines we must understand and attempt to eliminate the potential power relationship we have with clients, which, if unchecked, will obstruct the application of research in practice.

It is interesting that, in Jo Cooke's traffic-light project, the changes in attitude demonstrated by the adolescents that reached statistical significance related to ownership of the problem, i.e. empowerment of the adolescents, indicating that important decisions affecting young people should be made by young people and not by adults. Kate Gerrish and colleagues emphasized the importance of empowering both the clients that were served by Middleton NDU and their carers, and Linda Pearson pointed out that some of the best facilitators in participatory appraisal are the community members themselves.

Related to the issue of user involvement is the use of local data, which several of the projects highlighted as important (see Chapters 8, 9 and 10). Participatory appraisal is pivoted on user involvement and the use of local data to develop communities. In their chapters, Jo Cooke and Kate Gerrish and colleagues also emphasized the prime importance of addressing the needs of the local community.

OUTCOMES

Evaluation is an essential component of any development in practice. Evaluation can be carried out at the end of the project – summative evaluation – or throughout, to inform the course of the project (see Chapter 5). When developing practice in the community, it often makes more sense to carry out evaluation throughout the project. Jo Cooke's project provided an example of the use of formative evaluation in a repeating cycle of stopping, thinking and acting; she emphasized the importance of evaluating in a way that is reflective and continuous. Another good example of this is found in participatory appraisal, where evaluation is also carried out throughout the project through the repeated questioning of the process. Kate Gerrish and colleagues made the point that if the final evaluation of a project is favourable, the work should continue, which may not happen as a matter of course. This group found that other community nursing colleagues were sometimes reluctant to adopt innovations in practice from the NDU. Enabling projects or local developments to become mainstream service activities may require strategies such as those discussed in Chapter 4. This is an area of practice development that probably needs further work – while teams may be effective in undertaking short-term practice development projects, large-scale change of the whole PCT, which will be needed in the coming years, needs to build on the evaluations and experience gained from practice development initiatives such as the Middleton NDU.

Audit can be a useful tool to evaluate a development in practice against pre-set standards. Joyce Marshall found that audit with visual peer comparison and feedback helped to identify where improvement was needed in the application of evidence-based guidelines to the practice of leg ulcer management. Visual peer comparison, in the form of graphs comparing the performance of practices, was a useful feedback mechanism and provided positive reinforcement to the teams.

Several of the projects used visual outcomes and methods, which can be powerful tools. Joyce Marshall recommended finding ways to do this. Jo Cooke's traffic lights were a helpful visual symbol: stop, think and do. She also used video clips, posters, soap-opera character card games and weighing scales. Visual tools are used extensively in participatory appraisal, as the many examples in Linda Pearson's chapter illustrate.

However, if the time scale is short, over-reliance on outcome measures can be a problem in practice development. For example, in Jo Cooke's project, only minor changes in coping strategies were seen, which might have been more dramatic over a longer period of time. This can lead to practitioners becoming disillusioned. Interim measures, for example the uptake of exercise classes or a change in diet as opposed to a reduction in weight, are important markers for change and also maintain motivation (*see* Chapters 4 and 5).

ISSUES ARISING FROM SPECIFIC PROJECTS

Certain issues that arose from individual projects were specific to that project, but offer useful ideas to practitioners embarking upon similar work. For example, Joyce Marshall found that the links that the district nurses in one practice had made with a hospital prior to the project, to learn about leg ulcer management, were invaluable. This was a quick, easy process that enabled them to develop the skills they needed rapidly and helped them to develop a greater understanding of secondary care. Joyce Marshall also found that critical skills appraisal training was very useful for enabling practitioners to interpret the research evidence they were being asked to adopt in practice.

Kate Gerrish and colleagues demonstrated that the NDU could be an effective way to develop practice and to provide nursing services. However, they acknowledged that it is very hard to evaluate an NDU as there is no comparison group. A useful measure of their success would be the adoption of their practices by colleagues from outside the NDU, but, as mentioned earlier, there was a certain amount of resistance to this. Jo Cooke also describes a project situation in which there was no comparison group and discusses a before-and-after study of impact of the educational intervention on the adolescents, an approach that could also be applied in the NDU situation.

Another lesson from Kate Gerrish and her colleagues is the importance of networking. NDU clinical leaders found it helpful to meet with other clinical leaders from NDUs. When we had been newly appointed to our practice development posts in Yorkshire, we certainly found that networking with other colleagues in similar positions was invaluable. Useful contacts for networking for community nurses engaged in practice development are found in Chapter 12.

Hilary Gledhill demonstrated that clinical supervision can be a useful mechanism for introducing change, as in her project which introduced clinical guidelines to minor injury units. This was a useful strategy to get an initially sceptical team on board and to discuss misconceptions about the use of clinical guidelines in practice.

CONCLUSION

To conclude, it is clear that anyone involved in practice development needs to be realistic about what can be achieved. Kate Gerrish and colleagues found that there was an expectation by others that the NDU would be constantly embarking on new project work. Practice development needs to be planned, implemented and evaluated systematically, and it takes time to do this well. Individuals and teams that are embarking on practice development need to be supported. As is evident throughout all the chapters in the book, change is not without its challenges. The members of the NDU found they were under a considerable amount of strain, which needed to be recognized to prevent burn-out. Practice development can sometimes be a messy process, as demonstrated by Hilary Gledhill's project, in which she introduced clinical guidelines to two minor injuries units. The process of clinical supervision that was introduced threw up all sorts of issues that they had not thought of and which had to be addressed before the project could continue. A series of smaller projects resulted from the larger project, which is encouraging, but led to a lot more work than was initially planned!

As mentioned in the introductory chapter, the dissemination of practice development work can be problematic for practitioners, and networking can be one means of supporting such dissemination. Joanne Dorsman, Nicki Whitfield and Jane Mischenko have disseminated information about the Middleton NDU widely by collaborating with Kate Gerrish and other colleagues who are academics in institutions of higher education. Primary Care Trusts provide another potentially useful opportunity to disseminate good practice in support of their clinical governance agendas. However, as we saw in the review of the literature on change in Chapter 4, simple diffusion of research findings informs but does not change practice – planned practice development initiatives are needed to do that!

Strong links between academic staff in higher education and clinical staff are invaluable in practice development. There are increasing numbers of lecturer–practitioner posts, which combine university lecturing with development work in clinical practice, such as the posts we held in Hull and East Yorkshire as professional leads in Health Visiting and District Nursing. These roles allow the university to access the expertise of practitioners, and vice versa. This is vital if courses such as the

Community Specialist Practitioner degree are to prepare graduates for developing practice, if academic nurses are to remain up-to-date with issues in practice and if practitioners are to become involved in research and publication.

It is hoped that by publishing this book we have contributed to the process of disseminating the ideas and experiences of practitioners and researchers in community nursing, and that you will be able to make use of these ideas and experiences in developing your own area of practice. Some of the key ideas reiterated in these chapters are presented in Box 11.1. As we mentioned in the first chapter, there is excellent practice development work in community nursing being carried out in isolated pockets across the UK. The challenge is to network with colleagues, to share good practice and to publish findings from such developments in practice.

Box 11.1 Lessons learned about developing community nursing practice

- Planning is essential
- Identify potential barriers
- Identify your resources
- Secure the support of the organization
- Search the literature and critique the evidence
- Appoint a facilitator
- Use networking at all stages
- Include all staff from the outset
- Work as a team
- Involve and empower users and carers
- Address the needs of the local community
- Evaluate!
- Use visual tools where possible
- Set clear goals and outcomes
- Be prepared for other change stimulated by the practice development
- Be realistic
- Disseminate

Section 4

12

Resources

In this section you will find information on resources that will provide assistance with practice development. Web addresses frequently change, and therefore we recommend that if you cannot find a site using the address given here, you should enter the name of the organization into a general search engine to locate its present site, or use one of the health portals such as OMNI, TRIAGE or Trip (see below).

ATTRACT

http://www.attract.wales.nhs.uk

This web-based resource was set up in response to the needs of practitioners in primary care in South Wales. Individuals can log questions on the site; a rapid search is made for the evidence and a brief response is faxed to the questioner, summarizing the evidence. The results of the searches are also on the web site and include topic areas such as women's health, dermatology and general practice. Under general practice, for example, a question may be asked about the evidence of ways to help people keep appointments in primary care.

Audit Commission

1 Vincent Square, London SW1P 2PN, UK
Tel: 020-7828-1212
http://www.audit-commission.gov.uk

The Audit Commission has the remit to monitor public expenditure by more than 13 000 bodies. The Audit Commission publication *Change Here!* (*see* Chapter 4) is supported by an interactive web-based tool www.audit-commission.gov.uk/change-here and this could also be used to plan change.

Bandolier

www.jr2.ox.ac.uk/Bandolier

Bandolier is a print and Internet journal about health care, using evidence-based medicine techniques to provide advice about particular treatments or diseases for health care professionals and consumers. The content is tertiary publishing, distilling information from secondary reviews of primary trails and making it comprehensible. The internet version of Bandolier started in 1995.

Centre for the Development of Nursing Policy and Practice

School of Healthcare Studies, Baines Wing, University of Leeds, PO Box 214, Leeds LS2 9UT, UK
Tel: 0113-243-1751; e-mail: a.j.mcintyre@leeds.ac.uk
http://www/leeds.ac.uk/healthcare/consul/CDNPP/cdnpptoc.htm
    The centre provides an accreditation scheme for Nursing/Practice Development Units which is supported by a developmental programme for clinical leaders. It also facilitates networking of Nursing/Practice Development Units through the Practice Development Alliance.

Centre for Evidence-Based Child Health

Department of Epidemiology and Biostatistics, Institute of Child Health, 30 Guilford Street, London WC1N 1EH, UK
Tel: 020-7242-9783
http://www.ich.ucl.ac.uk/ich/html/academicunits/paed_epid/cebh/about.html
    This centre provides information on research, training and development concerning all aspects of evidence-based child health.

Centre for Evidence-Based Medicine

NHS Centre for Evidence Based Medicine, The Oxford Radcliffe NHS Trust, Headley Way, Headington, Oxford OX3 9DU, UK
http://cebm.jr2.ox.ac.uk
    The centre has been established in Oxford as the first of several centres around the country, the broad aim of which is to promote evidence-based health care and provide support and resources to anyone who wants to make use of them.

Centre for Evidence Based Nursing

Department of Health Studies, University of York, Genesis 6, Innovation Centre, York Science Park, York YO10 5DG, UK
Tel: 01904-435222; fax: 01904-435225; e-mail: health-matters@york.ac.uk
http://www1.york.ac.uk/healthsciences/centres/evidence/cebn.htm
    Evidence-based nursing (EBN) is the process by which nurses make clinical decisions using the best available research evidence, their clinical expertise and patient preferences in the context of clinical resources. The Centre for Evidence Based Nursing is concerned with furthering EBN through education, research and development.

Centre for Evidence Based Social Services

University of Exeter, Amory Building, Rennes Drive, Exeter EX4 4RJ, UK
Tel: 01392-263323; fax: 01392-263324
http://www.ex.ac.uk/cebss/sidenav.html
The centre has been jointly funded by the Department of Health and a consortium of social services departments in the South and South West of England, with the main aim of ensuring that decisions taken at all levels in social services are informed by trends from high-quality research. The aims of the centre are:

- Translating the results of research into service and practice development.
- Advising management on new initiatives.
- Dissemination of research findings to policy makers, managers, practitioners, service users and carers.
- Commissioning new research to fill gaps in knowledge.
- Working with training and Diploma in Social Work course staff to encourage greater use of research.

C.H.A.I.N. (Contact. Help. Advice. Information. Network for Effective Health Care)

C.H.A.I.N., Research and Development, Directorate of Health and Social Care –
London, 40 Eastbourne Terrace, London W2 3QR, UK
http://www.doh.gov.uk/ntrd/chain/chain.htm
C.H.A.I.N. is a network designed to facilitate links between health care professionals, teachers, managers, librarians, specialists, researchers and other professionals working in the NHS family of organizations. The purpose of the network is to enable members from different organizations, professions and levels of involvement to identify and make contact with one another. C.H.A.I.N. is part of the NHS R&D programme and disseminates targeted information, for example, on research findings or bids, via an e-mail list. It also maintains a resource of members' interests to enable collaboration on R&D activities by members.

Clinical Governance Bulletin

Clinical Governance Bulletin, Publications and Subscription Department, The Royal Society of Medicine Press Ltd, PO Box 9002, London W1A 0ZA, UK
Tel: 020-7290-2927/8; fax: 020-7290-2929; e-mail: rsmjournals@rsm.ac.uk
http://www.rsm.ac.uk/pub/cgb.htm
This publication is produced by the Royal Society of Medicine and is aimed at clinicians and managers in the NHS. The bulletins are concerned with communicating practical examples, pooling shared experience and highlighting and disseminating best practice in relation to the clinical governance agenda. Each issue focuses on a different topic, including: effective teamwork and learning; communication and clinical effectiveness. The bulletins contain short articles that are practically focused. The publication is funded by the Department of Health and is free to all those in the NHS.

The Clinical Governance Research and Development Unit

Department of General Practice, University of Leicester, Leicester General Hospital, Gwendolen Road, Leicester LE5 4PW, UK
Tel: 0116-258-4873; fax: 0116-258-4982; e-mail: cgrdu@le.ac.uk
http://omni.ac.uk/whatsnew/detail/1092850.html
http://www.le.ac.uk:80/clininaudit
   The Clinical Governance Research and Development Unit (CGRDU) came into existence on 1 April 1999. CGRDU succeeds and builds on the achievements of the highly successful Eli Lilly National Clinical Audit Centre. Since 1992, the Eli Lilly Audit Centre was a national resource in the field of clinical audit, particularly in the setting of primary health care and at the interface between primary and secondary care.
   Clinical governance, a framework for improving and accounting for quality of care, is central to recent UK government health policy. The CGRDU's principal function is R&D within the emerging field of clinical governance. Although there will be a continuing need to research audit methodologies and produce evidence-based audit protocols, additional innovatory activities are required to assist the successful introduction and continuing development of clinical governance.

Cochrane Centre

Summertown Pavilion, Middle Way, Summertown, Oxford OX2 7LG, UK
http://www.cochrane.org/

Cochrane Library

UpdateSoftware, PO Box 696, Oxford OX2 7YX, UK
Tel: 01865-513902; fax: 01865-516918
   The Cochrane Library is an electronic publication designed to supply high-quality evidence to inform people providing and receiving care and those responsible for research, teaching, funding and administration at all levels. Cochrane databases of interest to community nurses comprise the Cochrane Database of Systematic Reviews, the Database of Abstracts of Reviews of Effectiveness (DARE), the Cochrane Controlled Trials Register (CCTR) and the Health Technology Assessment Database.
   Most medical libraries subscribe to the Cochrane Library and it can be accessed on the Internet via, for example, OMNI (see below).

Community Hospitals Association

http://www.commhosp.org/objectives.htm
   This association has a number of aims, including:

- to encourage the improvement and extension of services provided by community hospitals;

- to promote, assist and co-ordinate education and research in community hospitals;
- to foster and develop strong links between the association, member hospitals and the communities they serve.

The association may be reached via the web site given above.

Community Practitioners' and Health Visitors' Association

40 Bermondsey Street, London SE1 3UD, UK
Tel: 020-7939-7053; fax: 020-7403-2976
http://www.msfcphva.org

The CPHVA has a number of special interest groups and other initiatives to provide support for members to develop and enhance all aspects of health visiting, school nursing, community and public health practice.

The Community Development Interest Group is part of the Community Practitioners' and Health Visitors' Association (CPHVA) and affiliated to other public health and community development associations (contact: Marion Hamilton, Community Development Interest Group Membership Secretary, c/o CPHVA, 40 Bermondsey Street, London SE1 3UD, UK).

The CPHVA Clinical Effectiveness support is provided via the Clinical Effectiveness Bulletins, the CPHVA web site and the publication *Clinical Effectiveness – A Practical Guide for Community Nurses*. The bulletins are published in the journal *Community Practitioner* and provide information on evidence in a particular area, for example parenting (Issue 6), training for effective practice, web sites and other resources. The book, Adams C 2000 *Clinical Effectiveness – A Practical Guide for Community Nurses*, is available from the CPHVA.

The Consumers in NHS Research Support Unit

Consumerism NHS Research Support Unit, Wessex House, Upper Market Street, Eastleigh, Hampshire SO50 9FD
Tel: 023 8065 1088; e-mail: admin@conres.co.uk
http://www.conres.co.uk/

This organization is funded by the NHS R&D budget. It helps researchers to incorporate user perspectives in their work and is a valuable source of reports and networks for people involved in participatory research. In addition, the unit commissions and undertakes research about the involvement of consumers in health research; produces publications and reports, and organizes seminars, conferences and workshops on consumer involvement in health research.

Critical Appraisal Skills Programme (CASP)

Institute of Health Sciences, Old Road, Headington, Oxford OX3 7LF, UK
Tel: 01865-226669; fax: 01865-226959
http://www.phru.org.uk/~casp/index.htm

CASP helps people develop the skills they need to appraise evidence affecting health. The aim is to enable decision makers, and those who seek to influence them, to acquire the skills to make sense of, and act on, the evidence. In addition to running workshops on critical appraisal, CASP runs train-the-trainer workshops and the CASP network of local co-ordinators and people with specialist areas of practice.

Department of Health

Richmond House, 79 Whitehall, London SW1A 2NS, UK
Tel: 0207-210-4850 (line open from 10.00 to 17.00 Monday to Friday); e-mail: dhmail@doh.gsi.gov.uk
http://www.doh.gov.uk

This site gives you the latest news and information about the department and its work. It also offers you easy access to the wide range of publications, policy and guidance produced. The What's New page is a useful resource. There are Social Care and Public Health pages that are of interest to community nurses. The site also offers useful links to other relevant sites.

Almost all the material published by the Department of Health is accessible in electronic format. Useful starting places for new visitors are POINT (Publications on the Internet) and COIN (Circulars on the Internet).

Effective Health Care bulletins

http://www.york.ac.uk/inst/crd/ehcb.htm

The full text of the bulletins is available on this web site and can be downloaded from the site. Each bulletin examines the effectiveness of a health care intervention. The bulletins are based on systematic reviews and synthesis of research on the clinical effectiveness, cost-effectiveness and acceptability of interventions. The bulletins summarize the reviews and provide recommendations for practice, and further research, based on the assessment of the research reviewed.

Effectiveness Matters

http://www.york.ac.uk/inst/crd/em.htm

Effectiveness Matters is produced to complement *Effective Health Care*, and provides updates on the effectiveness of important health interventions for practitioners and decision makers in the NHS. It covers topics in a shorter and more journalistic style, summarizing the results of high-quality systematic reviews.

Both *Effective Health Care* and *Effectiveness Matters* are subject to extensive and rigorous peer review. Over 90 000 copies of *Effectiveness Matters* are distributed free within the NHS in a similar way to *Effective Health Care*. However, *Effectiveness Matters* is distributed directly to GPs in England.

Evidence-Based Nursing

http://www.evidencebasednursing.com

Launched in 1998, the purpose of the journal *Evidence-Based Nursing* is to alert practising nurses to important and clinically relevant advances in treatment (including specific interventions and systems of care), diagnosis, aetiology, prognosis/outcome research, quality improvement, continuing education, economic evaluation and qualitative research. This is done by selecting original and review articles, the results of which are most likely to be accurate and clinically useful.

Evidence-Based Medicine

http://ebm.bmjjournals.com/
   This journal provides information on all aspects of evidence-based practice in medicine. The website provides information on the contents of the current issue, useful links to other sites, access to Medline and other helpful resources.

The Foundation of Nursing Studies

32 Buckingham Palace Road, London SW1W 0RE, UK
Tel: 020-7233-5750
http://www.fons.org
   The Foundation of Nursing Studies was established in 1991 with the prime aim of providing support to nurses to implement research findings and improve patient care. The Foundation: supports nurses; promotes evidence-based practice to improve patient care; makes nursing research and evidence accessible, understandable and relevant.
   The Practice Development Forum within the Foundation brings together nurses working in practice development. The main aims of the Forum include encouraging collaborative, evidence-based practice development, facilitating clinical effectiveness and contributing to the direction of local and national agendas.

Guidelines Sites

http://www.nice.org.uk
   A useful source of guidelines is found at the NICE website. NICE guidelines are based on the best available research evidence and professional advice. They take into account both clinical effectiveness and cost effectiveness and must be practical and affordable. In developing guidelines, NICE involves the clinical professions in the NHS and those who speak for patients. NICE guidelines may be developed from existing clinical guidelines prepared by others if they fulfil the NICE criteria for quality and content. Or NICE may commission new guidelines from start to finish. Research may be commissioned by NICE or guidelines may consist of existing material.
   Another useful resource is the American National Guidelines Clearing House. The NGC is a comprehensive database of evidence-based clinical practice guidelines and related documents produced by the Agency for Healthcare Research and Quality (AHRQ) formerly the Agency for Health Care Policy and Research (AHCPR). It can be found online at:
http://www.guideline.gov

Health Action Zones

Health Development Agency, Trevelyan House, 30 Great Peter Street, London SW1P 2HW, UK
Enquiry line: 020-7413-1994
http://www.haznet.org.uk
HAZnet was launched in 1999 in response to requests from Health Action Zones themselves. HAZs identified a need for collaboration, discussion and information sharing between each other despite their geographical differences and their unique local identities and objectives. HAZnet uses web technology to respond to this need, enabling people interested and involved in HAZs to communicate online.

Health Development Agency

Trevelyan House, 30 Great Peter Street, London SW1P 2HW, UK
http://www.hda-online.org.uk/
The Health Development Agency is a special health authority working to improve the health of communities in England with a particular focus on the reduction of health inequalities. In partnership with others, it gathers evidence of what works, advises on standards, for example in relation to education of public health practitioners, and contributes to the development of the skills of those working to improve people's health. The Agency collates evidence concerning a large number of issues, including the health of children, obesity, smoking, community development. The Agency also maintains a number of informative web sites. The Health Development Agency produces a range of publications, including *Health Development Today* which may be obtained from the Agency or is available on the web site and provides news and information on public health issues.

The Health Visitor and School Nurse Innovations Network

Centre for Innovation in Primary Care, Walsh Court, 10 Bells Square, Sheffield S1 2FY, UK
Tel: 0114-220-2007; fax: 0114-220-2001; e-mail: cipc@innovate.org.uk
http://www.innovate.org.uk
This network is maintained by the Centre for Innovation in Primary Care and has the following aims: to provide a directory of innovative practice in health visiting and school nursing from across the UK; to provide an electronic discussion group; and to provide a human network to enable innovators in practice and potential innovators to get in contact with each other. Those involved in practice development activities can have information about their initiative added to the web site.

Hull Developing our Communities

Hull DOC, 124/5 Highcourt, Orchard Park, Hull HU6 9SY, UK
Tel: 01482-854550
Participatory Rural Appraisal training, Tel: 01482-215503

Hull DOC is an organization in Hull which offers Participatory Rural Appraisal (PRA) training on a demand basis. Health professionals are advised to register for courses in small numbers so that group structure remains broad. A 1-week course currently costs around £350 per person, creche facilities and lunch are provided, and travel costs to placements within the week can be claimed. The course is accredited by the Open College with 3 credits at level 3.

PRA network: Hull DOC and another organization called Community Focus (Tel: 01482-616616) maintain a network of people who have undergone PRA training.

Institute of Development Studies

Institute of Development Studies Participation Group, The University of Sussex, Brighton, BN1 9RE, UK
Tel: 01273-606261; fax: 01273-691647 or 621202; e-mail: participation@ids.ac.uk
Web site direct to the participation group: www.ids.ac.uk/ids/particip

The IDS produces topic packs of information on subjects including health, sexual and reproductive health.

International Conferences for Community Health Nursing Research (ICCHNR)

Secretary: Dr A Ewens, Department of Health and Social Care, The University of Reading, Bulmershe Court, Earley, Reading RG6 1HY, UK
e-mail: R.M.Bryar@city.ac.uk

ICCHNR is a registered charity (number 1042880) the aim of which is to promote the dissemination of community nursing research and innovations in practice; to provide opportunities for those undertaking research and practice development to meet and exchange information. ICCHNR runs symposia and international conferences to achieve this aim. A newsletter is distributed to the members providing information about current activities.

Joseph Rowntree Foundation

The Homestead, 40 Water End, York YO30 6WP, UK
Tel: 01904-629241; fax: 01904-620072
http://www.jrf.org.uk

The JRF funds research and development activities concerned with social issues. It publishes reports and summaries of research funded by the Foundation. The publication provides summaries of individual studies and can be obtained from the Foundation or from the web site. Examples of studies undertaken and reported in this way include: Preventive work with teenagers: evaluation of an adolescent support team (June 2000); Social care in rural areas: developing an agenda for research, policy and practice (May 2000); and Links between school, family and the community: a review of the evidence (November 1999).

The King's Fund

11–13 CavendishSquare, London W1G 0AN, UK
Tel: 020-7307-2400: fax: 020-7307-2801
http://www.kingsfund.org.uk

The King's Fund is an independent health care charity focusing on the development of health care in London. The King's Fund works to improve the health of Londoners by making change happen in health and social care. The Fund also works nationally and internationally. The Fund gives grants to individuals and organizations and carries out research and development work to bring about better health policies and services. The King's Fund aims to develop people and encourage new ideas.

National electronic Library for Health

e-mail: information@nhsia.nhs.uk
http://www.nelh.nhs.uk/

The National electronic Library for Health (NeLH) is a national web-based information library resource for the NHS and the UK public. The library provides three services: access to a library of high-quality information resources, including The Cochrane Library and a database of clinical guidelines; Virtual Branch Libraries, which are independent online communities that create and share information on a particular topic such as cancer or mental health; and access to accredited online health information for patients and the public through NHS Direct Online.

NHS Alliance

Retford Hospital, North Road, Retford, Nottinghamshire DN22 7XF, UK
Tel: 01777-869080; fax: 01777-869081; e-mail: Office@NHSAlliance.org
http://nhsalliance.org

The Alliance acts as a representative body for organizations within primary care and provides opportunities for those working in primary care to network and exchange information on best practice. The history of the development of the Alliance illustrates its commitment to innovation in primary health care. Currently the Alliance represents three-quarters of the primary care organizations in England. The Alliance provides a range of support mechanisms for members, including a helpline, publications, a web site and regional and national meetings.

NHS Beacons Programme – Spreading Good Practice Across the NHS

Beacon Learning Advisors provide advice on becoming a Beacon site, Tel: 01730-235038 or e-mail: nhsbeacons@statusmeetings.co.uk
http://www.nhsbeacons.org.uk/main.htm

The NHS Beacons programme identifies sites of good practice across the NHS, for example in primary care and A&E. The Beacon sites provide a number of different dissemination activities to enable the lessons they have learnt to be transferred to others. A handbook is available listing all the beacon sites, and handbooks bringing together lessons from the sites are published regularly.

NHS Centre for Reviews and Dissemination (NHS CRD)

University of York, Heslington, York YO10 5DD, UK
Tel: 01904-433634 (general information), 01904-433648 (publications), 01904-433707 (information service); fax: 01904-433661; e-mail: revdis@york.ac.uk
http://www.york.ac.uk/inst/crd

The CRD produces rigorous and systematic reviews on selected topics and provides a database of good-quality reviews, a dissemination service and an information service in support of the promotion of research-based practice in the NHS. The CRD produces the *Effective Health Care* bulletins (see above) and the web site lists ongoing systematic reviews in addition to providing a list of all previous *Effective Health Care* bulletins.

NHS National Research Register

http://www.update-software.com/National/

The National Research Register is a database of ongoing and recently completed research projects funded by, or of interest to, the United Kingdom's National Health Service. It provides information on a huge range of research areas of interest to those working the community, and provides one source for evidence for practice development activities.

NHS R&D Health Technology Assessment Programme

The National Co-ordinating Centre for Health Technology Assessment, Mailpoint 728, Boldrewood, University of Southampton, Southampton SO16 7PX, UK
Fax: 023-8059-5639; e-mail: hta@soton.ac.uk
http://www.ncchta.org

The overall aim of the NHS R&D HTA programme is to ensure that high-quality research information on the costs, effectiveness and broader impact of health technologies is produced in the most efficient way for those who use, manage and work in the NHS. Research is commissioned by the HTA Commissioning Board based on priorities identified by six advisory boards. The HTA reports can be downloaded from the web site and include many publications of relevance to community nurses, including reports on pre-school vision screening (1997); home visiting (2000); and breast feeding initiation (2000).

NHS R&D Programme

Department of Health, Richmond House, 79 Whitehall, London SW1A 2NS, UK
e-mail: dhmail@doh.gsi.gov.uk
http://www.doh.gov.uk/research/index.htm

The Department invests in research to support government objectives for public health, health services and social care, as well as contributing to the government science strategy. The Department:

- works with services, the public and other parts of government to identify needs and priorities for R&D on health and social care;
- persuades other R&D funders to address health-related needs falling within their remits; provides support funding for this (non-commercial) research to be carried out in NHS providers;
- itself funds and manages R&D (not picked up by others) needed to deliver Departmental objectives;
- funds research capacity development (including in primary care), e.g. fellowships;
- supports synthesis of research and dissemination of research findings to users;
- utilizes research in policy making;
- contributes to wider government science and technology strategy.

National Institute for Clinical Excellence (NICE)

11 Strand, London WC2N 5HR, UK
Tel: 020-7766-9191, 020-7766-9123; e-mail: nice@nice.nhs.uk
www.nice.org.uk

The National Institute for Clinical Excellence was set up as a special health authority for England and Wales on 1 April 1999. It is part of the NHS and its role is to provide patients, health professionals and the public with authoritative, robust and reliable guidance on current best practice. The guidance it produces concerns both individual health technologies (including medicines, medical devices, diagnostic techniques and procedures) and the clinical management of specific conditions. Guidelines commissioned by NICE, health technology appraisals and referral practice guidelines are included on the site.

National Primary and Care Trust Development Team (NatPaCT)

http://www.natpact.nhs.uk

The NatPaCT was established following the publication of *Shifting the Balance of Power* (Department of Health, 2001) with the aim of supporting PCTs through the provision of organizational development support. A whole systems approach to development is taken, and the site provides self-assessment tools for organizations to identify their developmental needs.

National Primary Care Research and Development Centre

University of Manchester, Williamson Building, Oxford Road, Manchester M13 9PL, UK
Tel: 0161-275-7601; fax: 0161-275-7600
http://www.npcrdc.man.ac.uk

The National Primary Care Research and Development Centre is a multidisciplinary centre for primary care research. The centre was established in 1995 as a collaboration between the Universities of Manchester, Salford and York. The goal of the centre is to support service and policy development in the NHS by producing and disseminating high-quality research.

National Service Frameworks

http://www.doh.gov.uk/nsf/nsf.home.htm

National Service Frameworks provide the evidence base for the planning of health services to meet specified targets for health gain in relation to particular clinical need. Each framework sets standards and targets with time limits for achievement in areas including care of older people, mental health and cardiac health.

Nuffield Institute

71–75 Clarendon Road, Leeds LS2 9PL, UK
Tel: 0113-233-6633; fax: 0113-246-0899; e-mail: nuffield@leeds.ac.uk
www.leeds.ac.uk/nuffield

The Institute's mission is to contribute to the quality of life for users of health and social services through evidence-based improvements in the management and delivery of those services. The Institute seeks to combine academic excellence with practical relevance through integrated programmes of research, teaching and consultancy.

Nursing and Midwifery Council

http://www.nmc-uk.org

The Nursing and Midwifery Council has taken over the former roles of the UKCC and ENB. It carries out the quality assurance functions of the previous ENB.

Nursing Times Good Practice Network

Emap Healthcare Ltd, Greater London House, Hampstead Road, London NW1 7EJ, UK
Tel: 020-7383-5865; fax: 020-7874-0512; e-mail: gpn@emap.com

This network, which incorporates the International Midwifery Network, has four aims:

1. to stimulate and share good health care practice;
2. to encourage practice-based research, current knowledge and informed experience;

3. to encourage innovation in practice; and

4. to provide practical support for clinicians working towards these goals.

Full membership is open to those in practice or practice development, while associate membership is open to those not in clinical practice or to students.

OMNI: Organizing Medical Networked Information

Greenfield Medical Library, Queen's Medical Centre, Nottingham NG7 2UH, UK
e-mail: help@omni.ac.uk
http://omni.ac.uk
OMNI provides a gateway to resources on the Internet which are relevant to health care. OMNI's aim is to enhance the use of biomedical Internet resources for academics, researchers, clinicians and students in the UK. OMNI also provides training in use of the Internet.

PRODIGY

http://www.prodigy.nhs.uk
This web-based resource provides 'practical support for clinical governance'. The site provides evidence reviews developed by small groups of reviewers. Topics are prioritized and, if selected, the reviews follow a standard procedure to ensure that evidence from systematic reviews, guidelines and policy documents is included.

Queen's Nursing Institute

3 Albemarle Way, Clerkenwell, London EC1V 4QR, UK
Tel: 020-7490-4227; fax: 020-7490-1269; e-mail: qnil@aol.com
http://www.qni.org.uk/
The QNI supports the development and promotion of high quality nursing in the community. It provides a number of awards which enable practitioners in the community to develop and disseminate information about innovative practice. In addition QNI organises conferences, commissions research and works with a wide range of other organisations to promote community nursing. It publishes a regular newsletter which is available free to those on the mailing list.

The Resource Centres for Participatory Learning and Action Network (RCPLA)

http://www.rcpla.org
This is a helpful web site which includes up-to-date information about participatory events taking place and Participatory Rural Appraisal training courses.

Royal College of General Practitioners

14 Princes Gate, Hyde Park, London SW7 1PU, UK
Tel: 020-7581-3232; fax: 020-7225-3047; e-mail: info@rcgp.org.uk
http://www.rcgp.org.uk

The Royal College of General Practitioners (RCGP) is the academic organization in the UK for general practitioners. Its aim is to encourage and maintain the highest standards of general medical practice and act as the 'voice' of general practitioners on education, training and standards issues. The RCGP established vocational training in general practice, and supports the setting up of clinical guidelines for doctors, the expansion of research into general medical practice and the promotion of primary care. The web site contains, amongst other items, a listing of current meetings, conferences and other events.

RCN Institute

Royal College of Nursing, 20 Cavendish Square, London W1M OAB, UK
Tel: 020-7409-3333; fax: 020-7647-3435
http://www.bath.ac.uk/dacs//gold/about_rcn.html#rcni_contact

As part of the Royal College of Nursing, the RCN Institute benefits from the large network of RCN professional groups of nurses, midwives and health visitors who have a wide range of clinical specialisms. Through sharing knowledge and expertise, the latest developments in research and clinical practice development are integrated into the RCN Institute's activities. The Institute is a leading centre for practice development and runs short courses on practice development, which consider the inter-relationships between practice development, research and evaluation.

Staff working in the RCN Institute collaborate closely with other professional health care organizations and are also involved in a number of international professional developments.

RCN Research and Development Co-ordinating Centre

Dave O'Carroll, Information Manager, RCN R&D Co-ordinating Centre, Gateway House, University of Manchester, Piccadilly, Manchester M60 9LP, UK
e-mail: dave.o'carroll@man.ac.uk
http://www.man.ac.uk/rcn/

This web site has been developed to provide an easy-to-access means of sharing information on research and practice development in nursing, and is designed to be fully interactive.

The site will be permanently 'under construction' so that it develops in line with the needs of professional nurses endeavouring to conduct relevant research and to keep abreast of current activities in research and practice development in order to provide the very best patient care.

The web site provides a means for sharing information about research networks, policy issues, ethics, funding, training and support units, dissemination and practice development.

One area of the site is homepage of the Primary Care Nursing Research Network, which aims to put nurses, midwives and health visitors in contact with each other to assist in building a stronger research presence, amongst these disciplines, in primary care. The network runs an e-mail discussion group co-ordinated by Vari Drennan: v.drennan@pcps.ucl.ac.uk

School of Health and Related Research (ScHARR)

The University of Sheffield, Regent Court, 30 Regent Street, Sheffield, S1 4DA, UK
Tel: 0114-222-5454; fax: 0114-272-4095; e-mail: scharrlib@sheffield.ac.uk
http://www.shef.ac.uk/~scharr
Netting the Evidence: ScHARR Introduction to Evidence Based Practice on the Internet. Netting the Evidence is intended to facilitate evidence-based health care by providing support and access to helpful organizations and useful learning resources, such as an evidence-based virtual library software and journals (see also TRIAGE below).

Teaching and Learning Resources for Evidence Based Practice

http://www.mdx.ac.uk/www/rctsh/ebp/main.htm
These pages contain materials that have been produced to support the teaching and learning of evidence-based practice. The resources were developed for use in a 2-day workshop that was primarily targeted at nurses and the allied health professionals.

Trent Research Information Access Gateway (TRIAGE)

http://www.shef.ac.uk/uni/academic/R-Z/scharr/triage/
This extremely useful site is The Trent Institute for Health Services Research's gateway to hundreds of web sites containing teaching materials, tutorials, articles and other educational tools relating to health research. The site is intended to complement the courses run by the Trent Institute but should be of interest to anyone studying, teaching or otherwise involved in health research.

Turning Research into Practice (TRIP)

http://www.tripdatabase.com/
The TRIP Database searches over 70 sites of high-quality medical information. It gives direct, hyperlinked access to the largest collection of 'evidence-based' material on the web, as well as articles from premier on-line journals, such as the *British Medical Journal, Journal of the American Medical Association, New England Journal of Medicine,* etc.

Unit for Evidence-Based Practice and Policy

Dr Trisha Greenhalgh (Director), Ms Marcia Rigby (Administrator), Unit for Evidence-Based Practice and Policy, Department of Primary Care and Population Sciences, Royal Free and University College London Medical School, Archway Campus, Highgate Hill, London N19 5NF, UK
Tel: +44 (0) 20-7288-3246; fax + 44 (0) 20-7288-8004; e-mail: ebp@ucl.ac.uk
http://www.ucl.ac.uk/openlearning/uebpp/uebpp.htm

The UEBPP is a virtual subunit of the Department of Primary Care and Population Sciences (PCPS) at University College London. The aims of the Unit for Evidence-Based Practice and Policy are:

- To promote communication between the separate initiatives on evidence-based practice being undertaken in the department.
- To promote the multidisciplinary focus, qualitative and context-sensitive dimension, and population perspective of evidence-based health care, as well as the more limited paradigm of evidence-based medicine, which is perceived by some as being doctor-dominated and limited in focus to the individual consultation.
- To integrate the dissemination of evidence-based practice into the wider programme of education and development for local general practitioners and other primary care staff.
- To develop and implement appropriate training in evidence-based practice in the undergraduate medical curriculum and for junior doctors undergoing vocational training in general practice.
- To offer postgraduate academic training for primary health care, with a strong emphasis on evidence-based practice and policy.
- To identify, and pursue, new areas for the promotion of evidence-based practice in research, teaching and patient care.

Wired for Health

http://www.wiredforhealth.gov.uk
A useful website for school nurses. Wired for Health has been developed as a resource for teachers in response to *Our Healthier Nation*.

The WISDOM Project

http://www.wisdomnet.co.uk/
This web site provides educational materials to support health professionals in their life-long learning and professional development. The WISDOM Centre delivers networked professional development (NPD) for primary health care, using Internet technologies for information sharing and communication.

GUIDES TO USING THE INTERNET

The Internet and Other ICTs . . . An Introduction for Nurses and Therapists, by Carol D. Cooper

http://www.carol-cooper.co.uk/book/

This book is available only on the Internet and provides information in the form of book chapters on many different aspects of using the Internet, including the use of different methods of searching for relevant literature, sources of information on the Internet, different ways of presenting information to others. The chapters include many different types of activities which could all contribute to the development of the types of skills needed by those facilitating change in practice.

Your Health and the Internet by Dan Jellinek, Paul Lambden and Roy Lilley (2000)

Published by The Stationery Office, PO Box 29, Norwich NR3 1GN, UK
Tel: 0870-600-5522; fax: 0870-600-5533
http://www.thestationeryoffice.com

This book provides information on useful health-related web sites. It also provides a basic introduction to the Internet and advice about its use. The point is made early in the book that one-third of people who use the Internet regularly access a health-related site at least once a week. The book contains chapters on health promotion, resources for people with disabilities, medical publications and many others. Each chapter provides information and contact details for a large number of relevant web sites.

Index